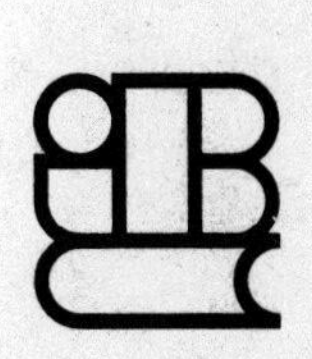

# Prison Madness

# Prison Madness

## The Mental Health Crisis Behind Bars and What We Must Do About It

Terry A. Kupers, M.D.

Foreword by Hans Toch

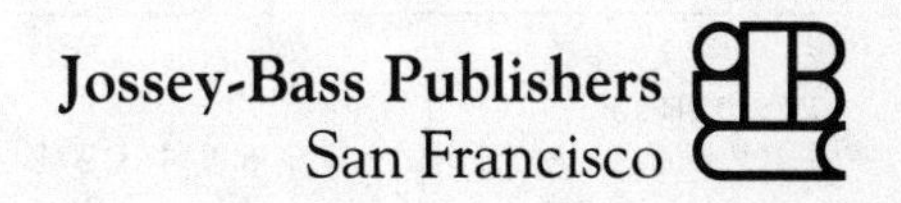
Jossey-Bass Publishers
San Francisco

Jossey-Bass books and products are available through most bookstores. To contact Jossey-Bass directly, call (888) 378-2537, fax to (800) 605-2665, or visit our website at www.josseybass.com.

Substantial discounts on bulk quantities of Jossey-Bass books are available to corporations, professional associations, and other organizations. For details and discount information, contact the special sales department at Jossey-Bass.

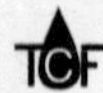

Manufactured in the United States of America on Lyons Falls Turin Book. This paper is acid-free and 100 percent totally chlorine-free.

**Library of Congress Cataloging-in-Publication Data**

Kupers, Terry Allen.
Prison madness: The mental health crisis behind bars, and what we must do about it / Terry A. Kupers—1st ed.
Includes bibliographical references (p. ) and index.
ISBN 0-7879-4361-4 (cloth : acid-free paper)
1. Prisoners—Mental health—United States. 2. Prisoners—Mental health services—United States. 3. Prisoners—Medical care—United States. 4. Criminal justice, Administration of—Health aspects—United States. 5. Correctional psychology—United States.
I. Title.
RC451.4.P68 K87 1999
362.2'086'9270973—ddc21 98-25505

FIRST EDITION
*HB Printing* 10 9 8 7 6 5 4 3 2 1

11/99

# Contents

## Part III: An Immodest Proposal

# Foreword

To be an observer of prisons is a delicate role, one that can be played in a number of ways, and also overplayed. Some prison observers play the amateur warden, obsessed with safety, management, and custody concerns. They are apt to mutter darkly about prison gangs, drug trafficking, and incipient riots, and to see prisons as beleaguered bastions of public security. At the other extreme are radical iconoclasts who view prisons as passing aberrations waiting to be abolished—though prospects of that, to be sure, are dim. Terry Kupers, by contrast, is a dedicated, persistent, and tireless but constructive critic of prisons. He is a humanitarian who seeks to ameliorate misery and reduce suffering that he feels is gratuitous, arbitrary, and unjustifiable, as well as dysfunctional and personally destructive.

Corrections is a profession and has responsibilities it cannot ethically ignore. It is one thing for prisons not to reform offenders (a goal now unfashionable to pursue), and another for prisons not to provide for basic needs of inmates, to fail to protect the vulnerable, to needlessly and pettily circumscribe, and, at extremes, to drive sane or mostly sane prisoners over the brink into madness.

Is the latter truly happening? Can it in fact be done? Kupers expends much effort to document instances in which the mental health of individual inmates has been impaired by neglect, callousness, and the impact of iatrogenic ministrations. In his effort to make this point, Kupers provides case materials in the shape of profoundly moving narratives. These narratives are a testimonial to the skill deployed to obtain them. It is difficult to elicit personal accounts in the prison, where feelings must be silenced and strangers treated with reserve and circumspection. To elicit biographies that convey suffering and despair, as do those in this book, is overwhelmingly hard.

It helps in this regard that Kupers has solid credentials as a principled advocate of prisoners' rights. His courtroom testimony has contributed to judicial decisions and out-of-court settlements that have improved the lot of convicts, at a time (now mostly past) in which prison litigation led to tangible prison reforms. As an expert witness in cases involving prisons and jails, Kupers had free access and unfettered contacts that few outsiders are afforded, and had credibility that few outsiders can acquire. If one combines these advantages with a practiced third ear and an awesome capacity for empathy, a predictable product emerges. This product reflects a perspective that is unashamedly and uncompromisingly liberal, and a stance that is unwaveringly humane.

---

The two subjects that Kupers deals with in this book—madness *in* prisons and the madness *of* prisons—are separable, but they converge on a central theme. More narrowly, Kupers is concerned with the adequacy of treatment of the mentally ill; more broadly, he raises questions about the sanity of specific prison conditions and practices. Both interests invite focus on instances in which indefensible correctional practices adversely affect the equilibrium of the vulnerable, whose hold on reality is tenuous or precarious.

The most topical case in point is that of the "maxi-maxi" or supermaximum-custody prisons, which are being constructed in indecent numbers across the country. These cold, metallic fortresses are touted as today's cutting edge in corrections. They are described by their sponsors as featuring the latest technology (which presumably is a self-evident virtue), being cheap to operate (what could be nicer?), and serving a critical function by housing the most unmanageable and troublesome prisoners in a system. Like most prison observers, I am myself nowadays surrounded by several supermaximum prison units in the process of construction. They are designed, according to state officials, "to house inmates who assault staff and disrupt our facilities," the point being "to remove (the inmates) from general confinement areas."

Given the concern about "removal from," there is limited interest in the point of destination, in the conditions of supermaximum confinement, or the fate that awaits prisoners who are shipped to supermaximum facilities. Officials acknowledge, of course, that conditions for these inmates are spartan and their surroundings austere. They mention—with a measure of pride—that their confinement means absolute confinement, that the prisoners never leave their cells except for exercise. They point out that there is no contact in supermaximum prisons—no human intercourse, at least—between inmates and guards.

What such statements do not convey is the extent of the sensory deprivation implicit in isolation of an undiluted kind. As Kupers notes, the experience entails spending months—sometimes years—in a monotonous, gray box containing a toilet, a shower (mostly turned off), a sink, and a cot, with access, for an hour a day, to a small wired cage. Tepid food is thrust through a slot in the door, and curt orders are barked over weirdly distorting speakers. Time hangs heavily and drags slowly in such settings, though some "progressive" supermaximum prisons offer self-study lessons through the slots in the doors or via preprogrammed television. Sometimes early release from isolation follows exemplary behavior—meaning, months or years of quiescence.

Kupers points out that supermaximum prisons (and disciplinary settings in general) become populated by emotionally disturbed inmates, since mental illness can inspire behavior that violates behavioral rules. Sometimes, a vicious cycle of symptomatic behavior and punishment ensues: Disturbed individuals who are unable to cope with conventional prison settings are often less likely to manage punitive confinement. The most extreme punitive confinement—such as supermaximum isolation—most heavily taxes limited coping competence, and leads, literally, to points of no return. Symptoms of mental illness proliferate, and prison cells become filled with prisoners who have withdrawn from painful reality and quietly hallucinate. Their symptoms, their torpor, incoherent mumbling, restless sleep, and waking nightmares are difficult (if not impossible) for casual observers to spot, and noncasual observers are unwelcome in punitive segregation facilities.

---

Prisons as such contain more than their share of seriously troubled persons. Crime is a no-skill, impulsive, disorganized, marginal game. We also arrest (thanks to the prevailing war on drugs) a share of the self-anesthetized discards of our stratified society, who are unemployed and unemployable. Such persons typically suffer from a variety of problems, very much including multiple substance abuse disorders. Moreover, it is obvious to most nonpsychiatrists that the line between mental illness and mental wellness is imperfectly defined by formal psychiatric diagnoses, so that certifying that a prisoner is not suffering from a florid psychosis does not tell us how stable or unstable the prisoner is, and how capable of negotiating life. Given that prison is a stressful environment, it is therefore unsurprising that the more stress we add, the more difficulties many prisoners will experience.

Ultimately, of course, the criterion for what makes a prison civilized is not the extent to which it impairs or fails to impair the mental health of prisoners. That would be asking too little of prisons, or any other institution that aspires to manage or take care of people (no matter how reprehensible they may be). A civilized human institution has to be decent and fair; it must offer its residents the opportunity to learn and develop; it must treat them with respect and must extend to them any trust or friendship they earn and any support and care that they need.

There are not many prisons that meet these sorts of criteria, but such prisons exist around the world. Someday, no doubt, a successor to Terry Kupers will write a book called *Prison Sanity* that will do these prisons justice, so that we can celebrate and emulate them.

*Albany, New York* Hans Toch
*July 1998*

To my parents, Edward Carlton Kupers, M.D.
(1909–1998)
and Frances Shirley Kupers, R.N.,
healers both.

# Preface

There is a major crisis brewing in our prisons. We are warehousing and mistreating a huge number of mentally ill people in correctional facilities, and many people are unaware of the ramifications. Others don't realize how current prison policies are traumatizing formerly "normal" prisoners and making them angry, violent, and vulnerable to severe emotional problems. Some people resort to wishful thinking while clinging to the foolhardy notion that the crisis can be contained within prison walls. In fact, the mental health crisis in our jails and prisons is already creating a public menace, and it will get worse. We are sitting on a time bomb. If we fail to defuse it, the consequences in terms of public safety will be dire.

Prisons and jails have become the largest mental asylums and providers of psychiatric services in the United States. The population of American prisons has tripled since 1980 and will double again by 2005 if current trends continue. As of December 31, 1996, there were 1,182,169 prisoners under state and federal jurisdiction and another 440,000 in local jails. Meanwhile, the deinstitutionalization of the public mental health system, combined with changes in the law that make it far less likely that a defendant's mental illness will be considered a mitigating factor when sentences are being decided, has put an unprecedented number of Americans with major psychiatric problems in the criminal justice system.

With the drive to send patients home from mental hospitals, the number of hospitalized mental patients has fallen from a high of 560,000 in 1955 to less than 80,000 today. In those same years, the proportion of prisoners who suffer from serious mental disorders has climbed to five times that of the general population. Between 120,000 and 200,00 prisoners suffer from major mental disorders, more than the total number of inpatients in noncorrectional psychiatric facilities. In fact, if all mental illnesses that warrant intensive psychiatric intervention are counted, including disabling but nonpsychotic conditions such as massive anxiety and posttraumatic stress disorder, there are more than 300,000 American prisoners in need of intensive psychiatric services.

Most prisoners afflicted with serious and long-term mental disorders not only receive grossly deficient treatment but also suffer horribly on account of increasingly harsh prison conditions. Understaffed correctional mental health treatment programs reach only a small proportion of the seriously disturbed prisoners. Many of the most severely disturbed prisoners are simply knocked out with strong antipsychotic medications and warehoused in their cells. The massive stresses and traumas of prison life worsen their psychiatric disorders, and their prognoses (long-term chances for recovery) become hopeless. Mentally disordered prisoners are called *dings* or *bugs* on the yard and victimized by other felons. Some withdraw into their cells, where isolation worsens their symptoms. Others strike out and wind up in "the hole," where they are even less likely to receive adequate psychiatric attention, and where the sensory and social deprivation make them even more rageful and delusional.

Harsh prison conditions have an extremely deleterious effect on the mental health of all prisoners. The large and growing number of prisoners who have histories of serious psychiatric disorders prior to their conviction are especially prone to break down under the massive stress engendered by overcrowded prisons. Many other prisoners, who never suffered from a psychiatric disorder prior to incarceration, react to the overwhelming traumas that punctuate life in prison by experiencing disabling psychiatric symptoms as well.

---

Consider the effects of massive prison crowding. New prisons cannot be built fast enough to handle the influx of felons convicted under mandatory minimum sentences and "three-strikes" legislation. Small cells, built for one, become home for two. Prison gymnasiums become impromptu dorms, crammed with hundreds of bunk beds. Over the same years that the prison population has exploded, education and rehabilitation programs have been dismantled, leaving prisoners with few if any meaningful activities and no opportunity to prepare themselves for "going straight" after they are released. The prisoners become irritable, tempers flare, racial tensions mount, abuse of the weak intensifies, there are more rapes, more men and women are sent to solitary confinement, and the rage keeps building. Is it any wonder crowding causes dramatic increases in the rates of violence, medical illnesses, psychiatric breakdowns, and suicides?

Prison constitutes meanness training; the meaner a prisoner becomes, the greater the chance of survival. Mentally ill prisoners have difficulty coping with the prison code: Either they are intimidated by staff into snitching or they are manipulated by other prisoners into doing things that get them into deep trouble. They are disproportionately represented among the victims of rape, they are extra-sensitive to the everyday traumas of prison life, and they are massively overrepresented among the prisoners in punitive and administrative segregation or "lock-up" units. Meanwhile, with the overcrowding of prisons and the removal of rehabilitation programs, the meanness goes unabated and proliferates, more prisoners crack under the strain, and a larger proportion of the population are locked in solitary or segregation units of one kind or another.

Instead of bolstering prison programming to alleviate these frightening developments, legislators and correctional administrators, afraid of being accused of "coddling prisoners," have opted to build high-tech supermaximum control units, replete with video cameras for constant surveillance and doors that open and close by remote control, where any prisoner who cannot behave himself or does not like the way the prison is run can be consigned for a very long time. Prisoners in these units spend nearly twenty-four hours per day in a cell where they are fed, isolated, and idle.

Keeping potentially disruptive inmates—those suffering from overt psychiatric disorders as well as those who seem relatively stable—in this kind of lock-up may provide a temporary peace on the prison yard, but a new problem emerges: What to do with them when they get out of lock-up? They will have had no educational activities, no rehabilitation or job training, no social interactions, and no training in anger management. And the conditions of confinement in "lock-up"— including sensory deprivation, social isolation, and total idleness—are known to induce intense rage and disorientation in anyone who is confined there, but especially in those who are prone to emotional breakdowns. In all the supermaximum security units I have toured, between one-third and half of the prisoners suffer from a serious mental disorder. Prisoners in these units who are prone to psychiatric disturbances experience an intensification of their hallucinations, delusions, and anxiety-verging-on-terror. Even some very large, mean-looking prisoners have let me see the terror in their eyes.

There is a move afoot to privatize the prisons. I am very wary, for reasons I explain in Chapter Eleven. Although it is true that state bureaucracies are prone to predictable inefficiencies and are unable to prevent many kinds of abuse, private, for-profit companies have a financial interest in thinning mental health staffs and lengthening prisoners' terms. With a smaller payroll (for instance, when psychiatrists take calls from home instead of showing up at the prison to work a shift) and more prisoners in the contracted facilities, profits grow. But this built-in self-interest in inmates' failure makes the privatization of prisons a very dangerous venture.

In the past two decades the courts have been looking into prisoners' complaints about overcrowding, harsh prison conditions, unfair disciplinary procedures, brutality on the part of guards, unreasonably long consignment to lock-up under extremely stressful conditions, and inadequate medical and psychiatric services. The bottom line in these cases is whether harsh prison conditions harm prisoners sufficiently to constitute a constitutional or human rights violation, and whether the psychiatric services are adequate to provide mentally disturbed prisoners their right to treatment.

---

I have served as a psychiatric expert in more than a dozen class action lawsuits concerning the conditions of confinement in jails and prisons and the quality of health and mental health care "inside." I have also served as a consultant to the Civil Rights Division of the U.S. Department of Justice and to Human Rights Watch in the course of their investigations of state prison systems. These roles have provided me an opportunity that is rare for someone who does not actually work "inside": entry into prisons, including interviews with prisoners, wardens, and staff.

I am repeatedly horrified by the degree of violence I witness or hear about in today's prisons, including violence between prisoners, assaults by prisoners on guards, and beatings and shootings of prisoners by guards. And when I tour the prisons, especially the security housing units where prisoners are isolated in their cells twenty-two or twenty-three hours each day, I am shocked to see a degree of psychosis—including inmates reduced to screaming obscenities, cutting themselves, and smearing feces—the likes of which I have never seen anywhere else in twenty-five years of clinical practice.

Willie is one of the many overtly psychotic prisoners I have met in prison supermaximum security units. (Names have been changed in most cases in the interest of confidentiality.) At fifteen he was tried as an adult, convicted of three felony counts, and sent to prison. He and another boy had kidnapped three women at knife-point while trying to escape from a locked psychiatric unit in 1993. Like many felons, Willie had been severely abused as a boy. At age nine, while he was taking care of his younger sister at a carnival, she was kidnapped and murdered. He never recovered from that loss and blamed himself incessantly. Soon after his sister's death he began tossing rocks at vehicles from expressway overpasses, throwing eggs at houses, setting small fires, running away from home, and being truant from school. He made several serious suicide attempts and was very assaultive toward other children and teachers. In his early teen years he was diagnosed "paranoid schizophrenic" and "mentally retarded," and was treated with Haldol, a high-potency antipsychotic medication. He was placed on the locked ward because he was considered very dangerous to himself and others. Even while taking Haldol, he constantly heard voices commanding him to attack people, especially women.

Even though Willie committed the crimes while he was clearly psychotic and attempting to escape from a mental hospital, he was charged with eight felony counts. In the course of plea bargaining, five of the more serious felony charges were dropped and he was eventually found guilty of three relatively minor charges. The verdict was guilty *and* mentally ill. The judge, believing that this fifteen-year-old mentally disordered and mentally retarded boy was a serious threat to society, sentenced him to several years in prison on each of the charges, to be served consecutively.

While Willie was in jail awaiting trial he was raped by several older prisoners, and the damage to his rectum was so severe he required reconstructive surgery. Nightmares and flashbacks related to the rape remain a part of his delusions and hallucinations today. At this writing, he has been in prison for over five years. In spite of his youth, severe psychiatric disability, and the fact that he was found guilty *and* mentally ill, Willie has received very little psychiatric attention in prison. He was transferred to the prison psychiatric unit briefly on two occa-

> sions, and he was given a prescription for antipsychotic medications. But left to his own devices, he quickly ran into disciplinary trouble and landed in the Security Housing Unit, where he is isolated in his cell twenty-three hours each day and eats all his meals alone.
>
> A psychiatrist and psychologist make rounds in the unit, but both merely stand in front of Willie's cell door and ask him how he is feeling. He reports that he never says more than a few words to either one because there is no privacy and he does not want the other prisoners to hear about his mental problems. He reports he sometimes sees devils lurking in his cell and hears voices commanding him to rape women and kill himself. Meanwhile, on several occasions he has cut himself very badly on the inside of his arm and across his neck. On other occasions, in response to hallucinated commands, he has thrown feces at guards. Each time he hurls excrement or refuses an order he is sentenced to a longer period in solitary confinement, which he says makes him even more crazy. Now it looks as though he will remain in the supermax unit until he is released from prison, which could happen as early as 2025.

Prisons contain some people who repeatedly commit violent crimes and deserve to remain incarcerated for a very long time. The public's understandable fears about these hard-core criminals should not be ignored. In fact, it is often these convicts who become predators in the prison domination hierarchy, preying on younger, less hardened felons, and making life miserable for mentally disordered prisoners. But contrary to the fears generated by media's concentration on the most depraved and violent, well over half of today's prisoners have never been convicted of a violent crime. If one tallies new admissions to prison rather than the composition of the entire prison population, the figure for violent convictions drops to 27 percent, because violent offenders serve longer sentences and accumulate in the system, whereas the large majority of prisoners are convicted of nonviolent crimes such as drug possession and other victimless offenses and released after a few years. Think about it, three-quarters of those entering prison today have not been convicted of a violent crime!

A large proportion of prisoners, especially those suffering from serious mental disorders, ran into trouble with the law on account of drug and alcohol abuse, and there is absolutely no evidence that locking people behind bars makes them less prone to substance abuse after they are released. Placing prisoners who were not convicted of violent crimes in this kind of hellish environment for several years only makes them angrier, meaner, and less caring toward others upon release—and the average prisoner will be released in less than five years. Ninety-five percent of all prisoners will be released eventually, despite the harsher sentences. Willie may eventually be on the streets again, and just imagine how much difficulty he will have complying with the most basic rules of acceptable social behavior after spending thirty years confined to a cell, hallucinating.

This book is about adult felons. I often mention young offenders. Everyone I know who works in the criminal justice system prefers working with youthful offenders, because there is more potential to turn the youth around and help them get out of the criminal justice system and stay out. I believe the emphasis of reform efforts should be on the youth, as I explain in Chapter Ten. Still, most of my experience has been in adult facilities, so that is mainly what I discuss.

Most hardcore, violent offenders are ultimately sentenced to life in prison. A bigger problem, in terms of public safety, is the much larger number of prisoners who are "sent up" for nonviolent crimes, mostly drug-related minor offenses. After spending a few years in prison, where they learn they must be violent in order to survive, they will have great difficulty containing their rage and acting appropriately in social situations once they are released. Whether prisoners are mentally disordered or not, they tend to come out of lock-up full of resentment and with a very short fuse.

In this context, I was alarmed to learn that the rate of second arrests (the rate of re-arrest for individuals who have already served one prison term) rose dramatically between 1985 and 1995, the same years we witnessed the demise of rehabilitation and education programs, severe prison crowding, and the advent of supermaximum control facilities. One-third of those sentenced to prison today are reentering prison because of revocation of their parole, and this is double the proportion of admissions that were due to parole revocations ten or fifteen years ago. The rising second-arrest rate and the growing proportion of parolees who are reincarcerated suggest that the imprisonment binge of recent years actually fosters crime and destroys ex-felons' chances of "going straight."

It is not uncommon today for a prisoner to "max out of the SHU." That means he or she is released to the community straight out of a supermaximum security unit. SHU stands for Security Housing Unit, but the initials have become the generic term for all supermaximum security units. There have been some high-profile cases in which ex-felons who had "maxed out of the SHU" committed very heinous crimes. Whether or not they all spend time in a supermaximum control unit, the prospect of a large population of ex-prisoners becoming more prone to commit violent crimes after spending time behind bars has ominous implications for social policy as well as public safety.

By portraying prisoners and ex-prisoners as potential dangers to public safety I am risking the perception that I agree with the people who claim that all criminals are dangerous and should be locked away for as long as possible. I do believe that what we do to prisoners while they are locked up can have very detrimental effects on their capacity to get along peacefully with others, inside or outside of prison. And I believe the effect is even more dangerous in relation to some mentally disordered prisoners. Mentally ill prisoners, like mentally ill people in the community, are not especially violence-prone when compared with other segments of the population. But I fear that the subgroup who are repeatedly traumatized and denied access to adequate psychiatric treatment in prisons, and are then sent to punitive solitary confinement units, do pose a danger to public safety after they are released.

I believe that heightening the harshness of prison life—by putting more prisoners in supermaximum facilities or by simply restricting their activities and taking away their weights and their law books—will merely drive more men and women mad. I will accept the risk of being misperceived as legitimating tougher sentencing in order to make a much more important point: The way we treat prisoners, with and without serious mental disorders, is foolish and dangerous. Alternatively, I believe we can institute programs that will help many prisoners shift paths and leave prison to become productive and law-abiding citizens.

---

Proponents of ever harsher sentences and an end to "coddling" argue that the high re-arrest or recidivism rate is due to the evolution of a new breed of incorrigible criminals or "super-predators." They say the solution to the problem of prisoners' coming out of prison meaner and more dangerous is to keep them locked up for still longer terms, even life. "Three strikes" and "mandatory minimum" sentencing guidelines fit the bill perfectly: "Lock 'em up and throw away the key."

There are several conspicuous problems with this approach, beginning with the gigantic public expense. The cost to taxpayers of housing a growing pool of felons and providing them with medical and mental health services is becoming astronomical. Prison construction has become a booming growth industry. And spending on corrections nationally has grown three times as fast as the military budget over the last twenty years. More than 600 new prisons have been constructed since 1980, at a cost of tens of billions of dollars. U.S. taxpayers spent $100 billion in 1994 on the criminal justice system. It costs taxpayers $100,000 to build each new prison cell. And the costs of construction are only the beginning. According to the U.S. Department of Justice, every $100 million spent on prison construction commits taxpayers to spend $1.6 billion over the next three decades to run the facilities. It costs more than $25,000 per year to keep each individual prisoner behind bars—or as much as $130,000 per year if the prisoner suffers from a serious mental disorder and requires psychiatric attention or housing in a segregated lock-up unit.

The financial burden is breaking the bank in many states and cutting further into already scarce resources for public education, health care, child protective services, road-building, and so forth. The state of California already spends more on corrections than it does on higher education, and other states are soon to follow suit. Keeping the population of felons who were originally sentenced for a nonviolent crime behind bars for life would require even more astronomical public expense.

No matter how many prisons we build, there is no guarantee that all criminals can be quarantined. It is impossible to identify accurately, much less round up, a "criminal element." A large proportion of crimes are committed by young men and women who have never served time in prison and who do not seem to be deterred by the prospect of harsher sentences. For instance, there is the replacement effect: Locking up the drug dealer on the corner is not likely to diminish drug traffic because a younger person will step in to "replace" the arrestee. This is true no matter how many inner city youths are imprisoned. But the whole venture is certain to create an expanding pool of younger prisoners. In addition, not all crimes and not all arrests lead to conviction, so that a great many perpetrators remain at large, no matter how draconian the criminal justice system and how much money we throw at it.

While the population of correctional facilities has risen sharply in recent decades, crime rates have remained relatively flat. Yes, there has been a fall of a few percentage points in certain kinds of violent crime in the last few years, but this shift conforms to a pattern of small fluctuations up or down in a relatively flat crime rate over the past twenty years and therefore cannot be explained by an imprisonment rate that has tripled or quadrupled in the same period. If imprisoning more people had the effect of lowering crime rates, we would expect to find sharp drops in crime rates in the states with the most rapid growth of prison population. In fact, a comparison of crime and imprisonment rates in the fifty states shows no correlation between rates of imprisonment and crime rates.

There is a self-fulfilling prophecy built into the logic of "law and order." When prisoners are brutalized and their psychiatric disorders left untreated, the rage they feel about their keepers' cruelty is interpreted by their keepers as proof that these "incorrigible criminals" need to be treated brutally. This self-fulfilling prophecy guides our social policy today. For instance, when governors and legislatures require a high prison occupancy rate before they agree to renew funding for operating the prisons, a huge incentive is created to keep more prisoners behind bars.

Large-scale imprisonment has very deleterious ripple effects. Everyone's constitutional rights would be trampled in the process of establishing the kinds of draconian measures required to keep even more offenders behind bars. Further, the communities from which the felons hail, predominantly low-income urban areas, are devastated by the mass imprisonment of their young men and women. The imprisonment of a significant proportion of a community's young adults can lead to family instability and foster social failure and criminal behavior in the next generation. A frightening example is the case of the two boys, ages ten and eleven, who dropped a five-year-old boy to his death from a fourteenth-floor window of a Chicago housing project on October 13, 1994, because the five-year-old refused to steal candy for the older boys. The fathers of both child-perpetrators were in prison at the time!

---

The majority of prisoners who are forced to spend their young adulthood in hellish prisons will get out, reenter our communities, and pose a more serious threat to public safety than they did before they were incarcerated. Because a significant proportion of prisoners suffer from serious mental disorders, it is especially foolish, costly, and dangerous to warehouse them in overcrowded prisons, deny them adequate psychiatric attention, and leave them to become the victims and perpetrators of violence. Most of them will also eventually be released. I do not say that merely to frighten the reader, I say it because I want the reader to join me in figuring out what would be a more humane approach to crime and justice.

In this book I will show you the horror, the injustice, the brutality, the senselessness, the incredible waste of taxpayers' money, the ineffectiveness and the failure of today's correctional system—for all prisoners, but especially for those suffering from serious mental disorders. Are the harsher punishments and more severe deprivations that are being instituted in today's prisons needed because the prisoners are more "mad" and "bad" than ever? Or are the harsh conditions, lack of adequate mental heath treatment, and severe deprivations causing the prisoners to become more violent, psychotic, and suicidal? I explore this question in some detail. I also offer a series of practical recommendations to reform the prisons, rethink the purpose of "corrections," and establish some guidelines for the delivery of humane and effective care to individuals suffering from serious mental disorders.

The book is organized into three parts. Part I focuses on the mental health crisis behind bars, and includes a description of the mentally ill behind bars and some reasons so many of them are in jails and prisons (Chapter One), a discussion of the traumas and stressors that cause so many prisoners, including many who have not entered the system with a prior mental health problem, to go crazy (Chapter Two), and a critical appraisal of contemporary correctional mental health services (Chapter Three).

Part II centers on the conditions that make prisoners lives so miserable and the mentally disordered prisoners' lives essentially unbearable. Its five chapters cover the psychiatric effects of racism in institutions where the majority of inmates are people of color and most of the staff are white (Chapter Four), some ways the experience of women prisoners is unique (Chapter Five), the ugly reality of prison rape and its psychiatric complications (Chapter Six), the importance of quality visits with loved ones if a prisoner is to do his or her time peacefully, maintain his or her mental health, and succeed at "going straight" after being released (Chapter Seven), and the recurring tragedy of prison suicide (Chapter Eight).

Part III explores ways to improve the plight of prisoners as well as the safety of communities. Chapter Nine reports on class action litigation that has improved the criminal justice system, suggests some worthy legal battles that are yet to be waged, and explains the ultimate shortcomings of legal remedies. Chapter Ten discusses the requirements for an adequate mental health delivery system and mentions some relatively successful mental health treatment and rehabilitation programs and recommendations for applying the lessons of these successes in all prison systems.

In Chapter Eleven I join the ongoing debate about criminal justice in the United States. What is or should be the social purpose of imprisonment? Is it simply vengeance against law breakers, or is there some hope left for rehabilitation? Will governments continue to withdraw financial support from education and social welfare agencies while expanding their corrections budgets? Will the logic of law and order drive us to continue "disappearing" the poor and dispossessed, or will we create a more inclusive vision of a better way to handle crime and respond to the mental health crisis behind bars?

---

I hope this book will awaken the public to some of the abuses and excesses I witness each time I enter a prison. I hope it will be a useful contribution to an urgently needed public discussion about the purposes of incarceration, what constitutes acceptable conditions of confinement, and how it might be possible to provide adequate mental services in correctional settings.

If we fail to take aggressive action right now to avert the mental health crisis behind bars, public safety will be in jeopardy for years to come. The prisons will continue to turn out enraged ex-prisoners, a significant proportion suffering from serious emotional disorders, who are ill-prepared to "go straight" and contribute constructively to community life. Many will be driven back into a life of crime. If, however, we stop the denial and open our eyes to the folly of current correctional policies, we will have an opportunity to alter our approach radically to crime and make a serious attempt to reform our criminal justice system.

*Oakland, California*
*August 1998*

Terry A. Kupers

# Acknowledgments

I have learned about the horrors and possibilities of prisons largely from prisoners and their attorneys. I am awed by the prisoners' frankness and their generous sharing. Many prisoners' stories went into this book. I owe them a debt of gratitude. I am barred from naming most of them, but a few individuals who do not mind being named have helped me a great deal, including O'Neil Stough, Horace Bell, Dan Pens, Daisy Benson, and Willie London. Raymond C. Walen and the entire Cain Gang, the prisoners' legal team in *Cain* v. *MDOC*, have even taught me how to be creative within the law.

The attorneys are a dedicated and courageous group, entering the prisons and struggling with wardens and attorneys general to permit experts to see what dark secrets need to be exposed. I have had the pleasure and honor of working with many very fine attorneys, including Terry Smerling, Richard Goff, Michael Satris, Don Specter, Allyson Hardy, Millard Murphy, Steve Berlin, Michael Bien, Sandy Rosen, Warren George, Luther Orton, Jordan Budd, Don Lipmanson, Carolyn Reid, Anita Arriola, Sandra Girard, and Charlene Snow. Jamie Fellner and Joanne Mariner, both associate counsels at Human Rights Watch, have provided me with excellent opportunities to see and to learn. Other prison experts who have served as valued collaborators are Craig Haney, Steve Martin, Jay Farbstein, Carl Fulwiler, and Larry Clannon.

I had the very good fortune of working with a talented and committed group of activists to put on a conference, "Critical Resistance: Beyond the Prison-Industrial Complex," at the University of California in September 1998. I learned a lot and enjoyed working with everyone on the committee, including Ellen Barry, Jennifer Beach, Rose Braz, Bo Brown, Julie Browne, Cynthia Chandler, Kamari Clarke, Linda Crockett, Angela Davis, Leslie DiBenedetto-Skopec, Gita Drury, Rayne Galbraith, Terry Day, Naneen Karraker, Stefanie Kelly, Rachel Lederman, Joyce Miller, Dorsey Nunn, Dylan Rodriguez, Eli Rosenblatt, Jane Segal, Cassandra Shaylor, Andy Smith, Nancy Stoller, Julia Sudbury, Robin Templeton, Suran Thrift, Ruth Gilmore, and Greg Winter. Other prison activists who are invaluable resources, collaborators, and supporters are Colin Starger, Noelle Hanrahan, Michael Alcolay, Corey Weinstein, William "Buzz" Alexander, Luis Talamantez, Christian Parenti, Michael Keck, Judy Greenspan, and Holbrook Teter.

Friends count for quite a lot. I find it impossible to write and do my work without the constant encouragement and interest of good friends. I won't name all the wonderful friends who have supported me while I undertook writing this book—they know who they are, and my hat's off to them—but I will mention a few who had to listen to me kvetch in the process: Richard Lichtman, Terry Day, Gale Bataille, Bill Berkowitz, Richard Hansen, Jeffrey Kupers, Lige Dailey, Franklin Abbott, Michael Kimmel, Larry Kupers, Don Sabo, Ram Gokul, Kay Kohler, and Peter Plate.

My three sons, Eric Guthrie-Kupers, Hyim Jake Ross, and Jesse R. Kupers, and my daughter-in-law, Kimiko Guthrie-Kupers, bring joy, inspiration, fresh ideas, and a reason to hope that the struggle will continue.

I can't express enough appreciation and admiration of my wife, Arlene M. Shmaeff, whose creative, social, and pedagogical ventures into the world enrich my life and my soul in countless ways.

Finally, I had the good fortune to work with a superb editor: Alan Rinzler at Jossey-Bass. He is a visionary with a wonderful way of showing a writer the right path for him, and a knack at keeping him on it.

# Prison Madness

# Introduction

I am often asked how a community psychiatrist becomes an expert on prisons. My evolution came by a circuitous route. In the late 1960s I served as the head physician at the Bunchy Carter Free Clinic in South Central Los Angeles, a community service program administered by the Black Panther Party (BPP). Volunteering at the clinic was an opportunity for me to provide medical care to a population that otherwise would have been grossly underserved.

At 3 A.M. on December 8, 1969, the police raided the South Central Los Angeles office of the Black Panther Party. They had heavy artillery and a tank, but the BPP members inside the office refused to give up until witnesses were present. The police fired repeatedly on the office until there were bullet holes in every wall. The Panthers eventually surrendered. Those who had been wounded during the gun battle were taken under heavy guard to a jail ward at Los Angeles County Hospital. They were handcuffed to their beds and surrounded by police.

I had treated some of these men and women in the community, and their families asked me to visit them at the jail hospital. The law entitled prisoners to visits from a personal physician, so I was admitted to see them. I observed the heavy guard. I observed what I considered unnecessary brutality. For instance, some of the wounded Panthers were handcuffed to their beds so tightly that the cuffs cut through the skin of their ankles and wrists. Meanwhile the police and medical staff were not very responsive to the wounded prisoners' complaints of pain or their pleas for medical attention. I was asked by the Panthers to report abuses to the press. There were headlines.

A few years later the Los Angeles chapter of the American Civil Liberties Union (ACLU) filed suit on behalf of jail inmates against the Los Angeles County Sheriff's Department, charging that the miserable conditions and poor quality of medical and psychiatric care at the L.A. County Jail constituted cruel and unusual punishment, a violation of the Eighth Amendment (*Rutherford* v. *Pitchess*, 1977). The lead attorney remembered my report about the shoddy treatment the Panthers had received in jail, and asked me to serve as an expert witness. At that time I was not very experienced in the assessment of jail conditions. I was familiar enough with related fields of knowledge, including research on overcrowding and the impacts of architecture on the residents of a facility. But this kind of jail litigation was new and would require a new kind of expertise. First I had to tour the jail and talk to staff and inmates.

There are fears connected with entering a jail, even for a professional conducting a court-ordered tour. Is it safe? The prospect of spending many hours rubbing elbows with prisoners evoked a certain amount of apprehension. I did not sleep very well the night before my first tour of the L.A. County Jail.

I remember that first tour. The smell of Chlorox and urine emanated from the "drunk tank" containing six or eight men who had been arrested the night before. There were "holding tanks" where sober arrestees were kept overnight, with little regard to who might be a predator and who a victim. There were the "rubber rooms," single cells approximately six feet wide by six feet deep that were "padded" on walls and floor. The padding was old, hardened, and in many spots peeled away from the concrete or metal underneath. There were no windows in the rubber cells except a small peep-hole in the door. There was no furniture, and a hole in the center of the floor served as a toilet, with the flush control located outside the cell. The men locked inside, some naked, could be heard screaming or pounding on the solid door. An officer explained that several of these men were dangerous, the others were suicidal.

In the holding tanks were men who had been in jail before and knew how to survive, as well as men who were in jail for the first time and were terrified of being assaulted. Walking along the jail corridors I heard the constant clanking of doors and barking of commands, and an occasional scream. It seemed to me that officers treated the prisoners with even-handed disrespect and inattention, as if they believed every inmate who asked something of them was merely manipulating.

The inmates' stories were poignant. As I walked through cellblocks and day rooms, accompanied by jail staff as well as attorneys for both sides, various inmates approached and asked who I was and what I was doing there. When I explained that I was a psychiatrist acting as an expert in a class action litigation initiated by the inmates, they proceeded to talk about their problems and ask for help. One man told of being beaten by guards. Another said he had been raped and needed psychiatric attention. Another cried as he told me his wife and daughter had stopped visiting and he was worried that they might be in trouble, or his wife might be seeing another man. He asked if I would be willing to contact his daughter and see that she was safe. Another told me he had a history of multiple psychiatric hospitalizations and asked whether I would be willing to do a psychiatric examination to determine whether there was a basis for him to plead diminished capacity in his upcoming trial. And another explained he would be released soon and would like to come see me to talk about the voices inside his head commanding him to kill himself.

The stories seemed sincere and believable. In fact, the inmates' stories were so compelling that I felt guilty for having to say no to most of their requests. After each of my first several tours I felt a mixture of sadness and relief, sadness because there was so little I could do to alleviate the pain these men expressed, relief because I was done, at least for that day, having to listen to their tales of woe.

After those first few tours something changed. It was subtle at first, and then it became more obvious. I slowly stopped diverting my attention from the specific issues I was being asked to assess—the adequacy of the exercise schedule or the waiting period before a prisoner would see a psychiatrist—to listen to the prisoners' queries. I began to quicken my pace as I passed the already familiar "holding tanks" and "rubber rooms." I became impervious to the noise level. I was beginning to numb myself to the overwhelming grief behind bars. In a word, I became more efficient in my touring. And the discovery that I was becoming numb in order to cope and do my job on a single day's tour gave me new understanding about the way jail and prison staff become inured to the inmates' plight. But later, after I showered and had a glass of wine, I noticed the shocked expressions on the faces of friends I told about my experiences in the jail.

---

The prisoners won that case, and the lower court's decision was eventually upheld by the U.S. Supreme Court. The consent decree guaranteed the inmates a certain number of hours per week of out-of-cell exercise, better quality medical and psychiatric screening at the time of admission to identify suicidal prisoners or those who might be suffering from a subdural hematoma (a blood clot in the brain) secondary to head trauma at the time of arrest, and significant upgrading of jail medical and psychiatric services. In the ensuing years I served as an expert in a dozen other class action suits concerning the conditions and quality of mental health services in county jails. In my tours of the jails in these cases, I passed many men and women asleep at midday on mattresses strewn on floors of dayrooms because the jail was too overcrowded to provide each inmate with a bunk in a cell. And I witnessed many other depressing sights and heard many sad stories.

After jail comes prison. In 1979 I was approached by attorneys to serve as an expert in *Toussaint* v. *Rushen* (1983), a class action lawsuit concerning conditions in the Security Housing Units (SHUs) at San Quentin and Folsom Prisons. At that time San Quentin and Folsom housed the toughest prisoners in California. (Many of these prisoners would be transferred to Pelican Bay State Prison when that high-tech maximum security unit opened in 1989.) The very toughest were consigned to the notorious "adjustment center," where George Jackson was killed in August 1971. At the time of my first tour there was a policy at San Quentin that all visitors must first go to the warden's office and sign a "no-hostage contract," which meant that the prison would not be held legally responsible for the visitor's safety in the event of a hostage situation. I was frightened. I began touring the huge cellblocks, each containing four or five stacked tiers of cells opening onto a huge common air space. There was constant noise and garbage-throwing, and armed guards patrolled along catwalks suspended in the airspace across from the cells. I had arrived in a high-security prison.

I have been asked at depositions and in court how I can claim to know about what is really occurring in jails and prisons when I have never worked "inside." I believe it is precisely because I have never worked in a correctional setting that it is possible for me to maintain some objectivity. Jail and prison staff too often become inured to inmates' complaints. Some admit that they have to tune out inmates' heart-wrenching appeals for help so they can get through their workdays and accomplish the tasks they consider priorities. Repeatedly, when I point out to a correctional psychiatrist that a prisoner I have interviewed is in acute distress or is severely incapacitated by anxiety or delusions, I am told there is nothing wrong with the prisoner in question, he is merely manipulating to get some attention. I begin to wonder whether I could be that naive. Or has the correctional staff become insensitive?

In one high-security state prison I toured I asked the chief psychiatrist about the incidence of rape. He told me that the press made too much of something that rarely occurred, and that no inmate had ever complained to him of being raped. In the several days that I toured that prison I heard of over a dozen rapes, reported to me by victims as well as perpetrators. It is possible that some of these men were making up their stories, but I doubt that. They seemed too sincere in the telling, and the victims' reports of ensuing symptoms were too like textbook descriptions of posttraumatic stress disorder. It seems more likely that the chief psychiatrist did not inspire enough trust in the men he interviewed for them to risk confiding in him.

In one class action lawsuit concerning conditions for the general population at San Quentin Prison (*Wilson* v. *Deukmejian*, 1983), I testified that the noise in the general population cellblocks at San Quentin was deafening, and proceeded to explain the detrimental effects of constant noise on an inmate's mental functioning. A correctional psychiatrist took the stand and disagreed, claiming that the men get used to the noise and cease to be bothered by it. During a recess the judge made an unscheduled visit to the cellblock in question, returned to court and stated for the record that anyone who thought that the noise level in that cellblock was tolerable could not be very sensitive to the inmates' plight.

I believe it is the continuing capacity to be shocked, or at least to be concerned when one ceases to be shocked, that makes a clinician capable of some degree of objectivity. I will share with the reader some of the cases and scenarios that continue to make me shudder, even after touring dozens of jails and prisons. Most of the stories were told to me by prisoners—a few came from published accounts, as indicated in the Endnotes.

PART I

# The Mental Health Crisis

# 1

# The Mentally Ill Behind Bars

A very large number of prisoners today suffer from a mental disorder serious enough to require intensive psychiatric treatment. But in every prison I have toured, mental health services are sorely lacking. A large proportion of prisoners suffering from serious mental disorders are ignored by the clinical staff, and even those who receive treatment do not get adequate attention. Except for brief hospitalizations for the most acutely disturbed, the average treatment is limited to medications prescribed during brief appointments with a psychiatrist. Meanwhile, guards punish mentally ill prisoners who cannot follow all the rules, and other prisoners stigmatize, victimize, or shun "crazies."

John, a thirty-five-year-old African-American man, had been in prison for seven or eight years. He had a history of mental hospitalizations dating back to age twelve, had been diagnosed as having bipolar disorder with psychotic features, and was taking strong antipsychotic medications when I interviewed him in the Security Housing Unit of a state prison. He told me that he believed the guards were singling him out for persecution, so he "bombed" one of them with excrement. They performed a cell extraction (four or five guards spray a recalcitrant prisoner with mace or pepper spray in his cell and then rush him and subdue him) and placed him in the cell with a plexiglass (lexan) outer door, where I found him. He also told me he suffered from hallucinations, did not relate to the other guys because "they would yell and argue," and he was "very depressed and extremely paranoid." It seemed to me that his disciplinary infractions were to a significant extent precipitated by his psychosis. It remains unclear what happened on September 11, 1997, but John was found unconscious in his cell and had to be transferred to a hospital where an inoperable, trauma-induced blood clot was found in his brain. He will remain in a vegetative state for the rest of his life.

---

Mary was hospitalized in a psychiatric unit with paranoid schizophrenia when she was twenty-three and again at twenty-four. When she returned home from the hospital after the second stay, she discovered that her husband had left with their two children. He eventually won custody. She fell into a deep depression, turned to illicit drugs, and stopped taking her prescribed psychiatric medications. Unable to pay rent, she became homeless. In the middle of the night, a police officer woke her and ordered her to move out of the park she had been sleeping in for over a week, and in the ensuing argument she struck him. Since she had two prior arrests for drug possession, the judge sentenced her to a prison term. I found her in a darkened cell in a women's prison in the middle of the day, and had to coax her to come to the bars to talk to me. She was quite disheveled and seemed frightened and distrustful. She told me she hears voices constantly but does not want to ask to see a psychiatrist because "all he'll do is lock me in a cell and make me take tranquilizers that make me numb and dumb."

In institutions where staff are unsympathetic and mental health treatment programs are grossly inadequate, the mentally disordered felon's choices are narrowed to two very unappealing options: to hide in his or her cell to avoid trouble, thereby risking depression bred of isolation, or to strike out when provoked and wind up "in the hole." This means a large proportion of prisoners suffering from serious mental illnesses are shunted into self-imposed or punitive isolation. Since their psychiatric disorder is likely to worsen under these conditions, and the large majority of prisoners will be released eventually, the misery of prison life has dire consequences in terms of public safety.

## How Do They Get There?

The prevalence of mental disorders among prisoners is quite high, at least five times the prevalence rates in the general population. Prevalence is the measure epidemiologists use to quantify and contrast disease occurrences, defined as the number of cases of a disorder in a population over a specified period. The period is usually a year, but sometimes the figures are calculated in relation to the total term of incarceration.

After reviewing a large number of prevalence studies, I have come to the conclusion that between 10 and 20 percent of all prisoners in state and federal correctional facilities suffer from a mental disorder serious enough to require intensive treatment during a single year. (The figure would be much higher if prevalence was figured for the entire prison term.) Comparable figures for jail prisoners are higher still, since many very disturbed offenders are incarcerated in local detention facilities for short periods and released without being charged, or they remain in jail only until a court has the opportunity to divert them to a treatment facility.

There are many reasons for the high prevalence of mental disorders within correctional facilities. I focus here on two very big ones: Number one is deinstitutionalization and reduced resources in the public mental health system combined with the criminalization of poverty, the net effect being more mentally disordered individuals on the street and subject to arrest; and two, recent changes in the law and in courtroom proceedings that make it more difficult to divert mentally ill offenders into noncorrectional treatment programs. In addition, there is a large and growing group of prisoners who had no psychiatric history prior to arrest but develop severe emotional symptoms after being stressed in a harsh prison environment beyond their capacity to cope.

## Deinstitutionalization and the Criminalization of Homelessness

Deinstitutionalization, the trend toward downsizing and closure of public mental hospitals, gained momentum in the late 1950s. At that time, Thorazine and other antipsychotic medications were widely available for the first time, and clinicians began to think about sending some of the large number of chronically ill mental hospital patients home.

With the passage of the 1963 federal Community Mental Health Centers Act, funds were designated for the establishment of comprehensive mental health centers in the community. Progressives in mental health called for a shift of funding from the state hospitals to community services aimed at preventing relapses and helping chronic mental patients live as fully and productively as their mental conditions permitted. But budget-conscious governors and legislators saw in deinstitutionalization a way to cut the mental health budget. They went along with the closing of state mental hospitals, but they did not follow through with funds for mental health services in the community.

An exuberant and impressively articulate patients' rights movement emerged by the late 1960s to protest the practice of involuntarily medicating mental patients and forcing them to undergo electroconvulsive therapy (ECT). Spurred on by the visionary writings of R. D. Laing, David Cooper, and others, radical therapists allied with patients' rights advocates and the resulting "antipsychiatry" movement campaigned against all forms of social control in the guise of mental health treatment.

By the early 1970s the war on poverty had ended, the federal support that had been meant only as seed money dwindled, funding for community mental health centers became scarce in the context of budget cuts and fiscal crises, and the plight of the mental patient, like that of the poor and minorities in general, was quickly forgotten.

Today, consumers of public mental health services are doubly affected by the downsizing of social service budgets: The safety net of vocational training and employment opportunities, housing, and welfare benefits is much weaker; then, when they find themselves in need of mental health services, fewer services are available. Since deinstitutionalization, many mentally ill people who would have been living in state mental hospitals or veterans facilities in the 1950s are now living in the community and lack the kind of support services and job opportunities they need to stay out of trouble. Individuals suffering from serious and chronic mental disorders are more likely, on average, to be turned down for jobs and then lose their homes because they cannot keep up with the rent or the mortgage payments. Some turn to drugs and crime. The incidence of AIDS among homeless drug users is very high. Not all or even a majority of homeless people are mentally ill, but a significant percentage are. And because some of them (but not all of them, or even a majority) have difficulty reigning in their idiosyncratic behaviors, they become objects of derision or they get into trouble. Today, mental health providers in the public sector are forced to tailor a major proportion of their services to the dually diagnosed (mental disorder plus substance abuse), the triply diagnosed (mental disorder, substance abuse, and AIDS), and the quadruply diagnosed (mental disorder, substance abuse, AIDS, and a criminal record).

Homelessness is not the only route to incarceration for individuals suffering from serious and long-term mental disorders, but I mention it as one example of the many ways individuals prone to mental disorders wind up behind bars today. A growing number of cities are passing ordinances that criminalize panhandling in city centers, sleeping on the street, and loitering in the parks. With the criminalization of homelessness, a significant number of mentally disordered individuals among the homeless run afoul of the law.

Individuals suffering from serious mental disorders are not known, as a group, for their capacity to control their impulses and follow orders. For instance, some of them fail to show a police officer the respect he feels he is due, and they are overrepresented among arrestees. Since they are less likely than other arrestees to have the financial backing it takes to navigate through the bail-bonding and plea-bargaining processes, they go to jail. Finding themselves in such confined quarters, some "fly off the handle," get into fights, and are sent to "lock-up." Others, more timid than mean, withdraw into their cells if they can, and fall into depression. Those who are not permitted to retreat into their cells become victims in the general population, where they are beaten, cheated, or raped by predators.

## Less Sympathetic Courts

Recent changes in criminal law as well as routine police practices make it much more difficult for defense attorneys to argue that their clients should not be found guilty because their mental disorder played a part in their criminal behavior. When police officers suspect that the person creating a public disturbance is suffering from a mental disorder, they can either take that person to an emergency room for a psychiatric evaluation or make an arrest and deliver the offender to jail. If the local psychiatric facilities are crowded (and, with diminished public mental health budgets, most are) and the officers expect that the troublemaker will be released from the emergency room rather than being admitted to a locked ward, they are very likely to make the arrest and cart the suspect off to jail. That way they will be certain that he or she will stay off the streets for a while.

Once mentally disordered offenders enter the criminal justice system, it is less likely than it once was that they will be excused from culpability or diverted into a mental health or substance abuse treatment program. Race is an important consideration in determining who will be diverted to a mental health treatment program and who will go to jail. White people are more likely to be treated while people of color are more likely to be incarcerated. Most low-income defendants in criminal prosecutions are represented by public defenders, who do not have the budget or the time to provide a thorough psychiatric assessment in every case and argue that the defendant had diminished capacity or insufficient mental competence at the time of the trial to be held fully accountable. In addition, many states have altered the rules governing the diminished capacity and insanity defenses, for instance by adding "guilty *and* mentally ill" to the list of possible verdicts contained in judges' instructions to juries.

When a jury is given the option of finding a defendant guilty, not guilty by reason of insanity, or guilty *and* mentally ill, the jury members tend to view the third alternative as an acceptable compromise. So a certain number of defendants who once might have been diverted out of the criminal justice system are now being sent to jail or prison in spite of their mental disorders.

## Breakdowns During Incarceration

Prison overcrowding makes life inside miserable for everyone, but especially for prisoners suffering from (or prone to suffer) severe and chronic mental illnesses. Rape is a serious trauma for anyone, but there is a subgroup of mentally ill prisoners who are much more likely than the average prisoner to become a victim (of course, it is also true that there is another subgroup of mentally ill prisoners who are more likely to be perpetrators) and to suffer a serious psychiatric decompensation or breakdown as a result of the trauma. Similarly, brutality on the part of guards and the shunting of a growing number of convicts into supermaximum security units make it even more difficult for prisoners who are prone to emotional collapse and suicide to do their time without breaking down or becoming self-destructive, even if they had no history of a psychiatric breakdown prior to being incarcerated. For example:

Charles, a twenty-seven-year-old African-American man, has been in the SHU for a year. He explained to me why he was first sent to lock-up: "I was being scapegoated by the other prisoners. I complained to the guards but they didn't take me seriously, so I had to throw feces at the guards to get myself removed from a very dangerous situation." Charles entered the prison system when he was eighteen, and claims he was not suffering from a mental disorder at that time: "I saw myself as antisocial all right, I'm very sensitive to rejections, and then I get mad and can't control myself. But I never heard voices or got paranoid before I got locked up in here."

In prison, Charles's sensitivity and lack of impulse control prevented him from getting along on the mainline (the general population area of a prison). Other prisoners would taunt each other, perhaps they would begin throwing things, and then Charles would "go off" and flood the range (tier of cells) by stopping up his toilet, or he would be the one to initiate the excrement-slinging.

Charles does not understand how other prisoners can "get rowdy" and then calm down when the guards come by and ask who started the ruckus. He is unable to calm himself. He remembers being "thrown in the hole" soon after arriving at the penitentiary. The other prisoners soon learned they could cause Charles to be sent to lock-up by taunting him and then acting innocent when the guards came to investigate. Once riled, Charles could not settle down, so he was always the one sent to lock-up. It was several years later that he began hearing voices telling him to kill someone. At this time, he wonders momentarily whether he is delusional but quickly reverts to insisting: "There has to be a plot, why else would I be the one who keeps getting in trouble even though other prisoners do worse things?" The pattern kept escalating until the guards began calling Charles "cuckoo," and he began throwing excrement at them. That was before he was seen by the psychiatrist and diagnosed paranoid schizophrenic.

Now Charles is confined in the SHU and takes antipsychotic medications. He tells me that the SHU makes his mental illness worse: "I can't concentrate. There's a lot of noise. Other prisoners are

> always calling you something, hassling you, all night long. It makes my voices worse, they tell me to kill someone. Sometimes I get depressed, then I do something ignorant like yelling back or flooding the range, that makes my depression go away even though I know I'm doing ignorant things."

Since schizophrenia and other major mental disorders usually surface during early adulthood, the age when most felons first enter prison, it is often difficult to discern whether a mentally disordered prisoner entered prison suffering from the disorder or the disorder was caused by harsh prison conditions and the massive traumas that regularly occur behind bars. I have found that the majority of prisoners suffering from serious mental disorders had a history of psychiatric problems before entering prison, but a significant minority, like Charles, had no such history. We do know that some individuals are more prone to psychiatric breakdown than others. The same kind of trauma, for instance the carnage of war or the horror of rape, will cause some individuals to suffer a psychotic breakdown. Other individuals will suffer the flashbacks and startle reactions that are typical of posttraumatic stress disorder (PTSD), and still others will not experience any significant psychiatric symptoms at all. There is definitely a relationship between stress and the occurrence of psychiatric disorder.

Even someone who has suffered at least one classic psychotic breakdown, replete with hallucinations and delusions, might stabilize quickly and suffer no further breakdowns if he or she lives in a caring residence and works in a sheltered workshop. But the same person, if homeless and repeatedly traumatized by assaults, will repeatedly break down and have to return to the hospital. Similarly, people who are vulnerable to psychiatric decompensation under severe duress might avoid breakdown altogether if their living conditions and social relations are adequate. But the same individual might suffer a massive psychotic breakdown if he or she is raped in jail, threatened with death for "snitching," or beaten by prison guards. This is even more apparent in cases of depression. Many previously nondepressed people become severely depressed in jail and prison, and a significant proportion go on to commit suicide.

Based on the large number of clinical cases I have reviewed and my interviews with prisoners and staff, I have come to the conclusion there is merit in both claims: A much greater number of mentally ill people are being sent to jails and prisons today, where their condition deteriorates on account of the harsh environment and inadequate mental health services; *and* the harsh conditions and brutality of life in prison are making previously very sane prisoners suffer psychiatric breakdowns.

## A Living Hell

For mentally disordered prisoners, danger lurks everywhere. They tend to have great difficulty coping with the prison code—either they are intimidated by staff into snitching or they are manipulated by other prisoners into doing things that get them into deep trouble. Women prisoners are less obsessed with the code, but they have an equivalent set of problems.

Male and female mentally disordered prisoners are disproportionately represented among the victims of rape. They are especially vulnerable to the negative repercussions of a lack of visits from loved ones. They are involved in racial incidents. Many voluntarily isolate themselves in their cells in order to avoid trouble. And they are overrepresented among prisoners in lock-up and supermaximum control units. To make matters worse, their plight is very often ignored by a staff that is singularly concerned about security and the possibility that they might be manipulated.

### Victims of the Male Code

The male prison code requires that a prisoner act tough. He must show other prisoners neither his fear nor his weakness; he must mind his own business, no matter what he sees or hears; he must act as though he is ready to fight if challenged, and early in his prison career he will be challenged to show his mettle; he must not do anything that might make other prisoners think he is gay, a punk, or a sissy; and he must not be seen talking to guards or staff in a context that might suggest to other prisoners that he is cooperating with the authorities.

"Snitching" is a capital offense. If an inmate protests that the weapon or contraband the guards find during an unannounced cell search belongs to his cellmate, he is subject to violent reprisals by other inmates; but if he refuses to snitch he is subject to a long stint in solitary confinement.

Mentally ill offenders have a very rough time coping with the prison code. Many find hiding their fears and their weakness practically impossible. For instance, while I was touring a high-security prison in preparation for testimony in a class action suit about prison conditions, I met a very depressed inmate who confided that he feared for his life. He was serving a prison term for fraud. He had played with money, other peoples' money (he was a financial consultant), and he had cheated. So he was convicted and sentenced to five years. But he was not very good at fighting with his hands, had never raised a weapon or been violent toward anyone, and he was terrified of having to be on the prison yard with "a bunch of toughs and rapists." He had never been depressed prior to his arrest, but soon after arriving at the prison he fell into a deep depression and tried to kill himself by slashing his wrists. He bungled it. Officers removed him from his cell and transferred him to "Ad Seg" (Administrative Segregation, a segregation/isolation section of a cellblock where prisoners are housed twenty-four hours a day and are fed in their cells—for prisoners who are being disciplined or are incapable of surviving in the open cellblock.) With severe overcrowding, the men in this prison are double-celled, even in the Ad Seg unit.

Because he tried to kill himself and the scars showed, this inmate was immediately labeled a weakling and taunted by others.

He refused to go out on the yard for fear he would be attacked. His cellmate was kind to him, even offered support. But some of the others within the Administrative Segregation cellblock began talking to the cellmate on the yard, warning him that if he did not beat up his "punk cellie" they would begin to believe they were lovers. At night, with the lights out, they would yell at the cellmate: "You'd better get that punk (the inmate who attempted suicide), or maybe you're a punk too." (A punk is a man who is sodomized, usually after losing a fight, or one who voluntarily becomes another inmate's passive sexual partner.) A few days later this depressed man was beat up by his cellmate.

Prisoners who are clearly psychotic and chronically disturbed are called "dings" or "bugs" by other prisoners, and victimized. Mentally disordered prisoners tell me that antipsychotic medications slow their reaction times, which makes them more vulnerable to "blind-siding," an attack from the side or from behind by another prisoner. And prisoners suffering from mental disorders are disproportionately represented among the victims of rape.

> Aaron is a twenty-three-year-old white man who had a long history of severe mental illness prior to his arrest and conviction for child abuse in 1996. He had been treated since childhood for a severe psychotic condition, and had been stabilized on Clozaril, a powerful "atypical" antipsychotic agent. He was happily married and the father of two children when his seven-month-old child stopped breathing while he was caring for him. The district attorney charged him with killing the child, and he was convicted and given a 100-year sentence. His psychiatrist, who did not believe Aaron was capable of harming anyone, much less his own son, was not asked to testify, but later said: "I believe what has happened to Aaron is a classic case of miscarriage of justice." In prison, Aaron, who stands five feet six inches and has a retiring personality, was singled out for abuse by the white supremacist Aryan Brotherhood as well as the Texas branch of the Crips. After he was taken off his medications by the

prison psychiatrist who had decided he did not need such an expensive drug, he began to hallucinate again and wrapped T-shirts around his head to protect his brain from hostile rays. His mental deterioration was quickly noted by prison toughs, and he was beaten and raped several times.

---

I interviewed another prisoner, David, in the administrative segregation unit of a high-security state prison. He is a slight, homosexual man in his early twenties who does not display any of the posturing and bravado that is characteristic of so many prison inmates. He was convicted of drug dealing, and because he carried a gun he was consigned to a high-security prison—but in prison, without a gun, his physical size and inexperience in hand-to-hand combat make him an easy mark. He explains that from the time he arrived at the prison, he has been brutalized and raped repeatedly—his overt homosexuality seems to pose a threat to other inmates, and they regularly single him out for abuse. He was told that if he "snitched" to a guard, he would be killed. He tried talking to a seemingly friendly correctional officer about his plight, but the officer insisted he give him the name of an inmate who had raped him, and seemed more interested in busting a guilty tough than in helping this man figure out a way to be safe "inside."

This prison does not have a Protective Custody unit. After suffering multiple rapes as well as serious injuries from beatings, David figured out that the best way to stay alive while serving his term would be to get locked up in "the hole." So he hit a guard and was sent to solitary confinement. He tells me he was not depressed before entering prison but has suffered from a severe depression ever since he was raped. He also suffers flashbacks and nightmares related to the rapes, severe insomnia, and an intense startle reaction—he jumps and his heart starts pounding whenever he hears a sudden sound. He cries as he tells me in private how lonely he feels, and how seriously he is contemplating suicide.

Another group of mentally disordered felons tend to strike out at the slightest provocation, and consequently suffer violent reprisals or spend a lot of time in solitary confinement. Whether they are victims or they strike out irrationally and get into trouble, mentally ill prisoners are poorly equipped to cope in the harsh prison environment.

## Women Prisoners with Mental Disorders

The plight of mentally disordered women prisoners is no better than that of their male counterparts, but the issues are somewhat different. The same social realities enlarge their number behind bars, including deinstitutionalization, poverty, cuts in social services, the criminalization of homelessness, the war on drugs, and changes in sentencing and courtroom procedures. Harsher sentences, especially related to drugs, cause overcrowding in women's prisons.

Although women are only 8 percent of the prison population nationwide, their number has increased by 275 percent since 1980, and they are the fastest growing subpopulation of prisoners today. There is very little educational and rehabilitation programming. As in men's facilities, overcrowding and relative idleness bring a rise in violence and psychiatric disability. And instead of solving the problem of crowding and bolstering the rehabilitation opportunities, correctional authorities in women's prison systems are resorting to supermaximum security units to control the heightened violence and disorder.

There is less violence among women prisoners than there is among their male counterparts. Consequently there is less victimization of mentally disordered prisoners. Women do not spend as much time as men obsessing about a code and "who's on top," and women are much more likely than men to team up and cooperate with each other in order to figure out how to survive their sentences. For instance, instead of victimizing sick prisoners, women often cooperate to provide the kinds of help the prison health services fail to provide.

A few years ago, prisoners at Central California Women's Facility sued the state, claiming that medical care was grossly inadequate. Charisse Shumate, the first named plaintiff in the lawsuit, suffered from sickle cell anemia. When a person suffering from this disease goes into a crisis, emergency medical attention is needed or she might die. One night, Charisse went into crisis, and began banging on her cell door to get help. No help was forthcoming. After several minutes, women in adjacent cells awoke, realized what was going on, and began banging on their cell doors in solidarity with Charisse. Finally, a male guard appeared on the tier, looked into Charisse's cell and hesitated. He was new at the job, and was not familiar with her medical condition. Maybe he was wondering whether this was just another "convict scam." Charisse showed him the copy of her medical file that she kept in her cell, but he said he was not interested in reading it. The other prisoners began exhorting him to do something, so he called the medical emergency department and finally Charisse was removed from her cell and taken to the local hospital. I have heard similar stories of collective support for women prisoners suffering from serious mental disorders.

Although the prevalence of all mental disorders in women's prisons is high, the prevalence of depression is especially elevated. In Chapter Five I spell out some of the special problems that confront women prisoners, including difficulties staying in touch with family, especially children. Since a significant proportion of women prisoners were sexually abused as children, and quite a few of this group have substance abuse problems, it is not surprising to find that many are depressed. Child psychologists tell us that girls are more likely to withdraw and become depressed after being traumatized whereas boys are more likely to strike out and get into trouble. The themes of childhood abuse, domestic violence, drugs, and depression are omnipresent in the stories of women prisoners who suffer from serious psychiatric disorders. For example:

> Sandra was sexually molested repeatedly by her grandfather from the time she was five until she was ten. She tried to tell her mother that she did not want to spend time alone with him, but her mother never listened. At ten Sandra began disobeying her mother, hitting boys at school, and getting in trouble with teachers. Her mother, an alcoholic who paid very little attention to her only child, gave her to a neighbor to raise. Sandra ran away several times, prompting the neighbor to send her to the adolescent ward of a locked psychiatric hospital. The psychiatrist decided Sandra was suffering from schizophrenia and prescribed antipsychotic medications, but he never uncovered the history of childhood sexual abuse.
>
> Sandra remained in the hospital until she was eighteen. She left to live on her own. She stopped taking the medication and began to drink heavily. When she drank she became belligerent. Whenever a male stranger annoyed her while she was drinking, she would hit him. On two occasions she was taken to the county psychiatric hospital, admitted, and given injections of antipsychotic medications. Each time she left the hospital she immediately discontinued the medications and began drinking again. At nineteen she slugged the police officer who was called because she was acting too rowdy in a bar. She was arrested and sent to jail. After several more incidents of this kind, Sandra was convicted of assaulting a man in a bar and was given a term of three years in prison.
>
> In prison, when she believed another prisoner was out to get her, she sought out that prisoner and attacked her. She was punished with a term in the administrative lock-up unit, where I met her. She appeared disheveled and admitted she heard voices commanding her to hit other prisoners. She told me she had never received any psychiatric treatment in prison, but she believed the guards were harassing her. She said they often walked by her cell whispering that another prisoner a few cells away was out to get her. She continued:

"Telling me that makes my face get all red and I start screaming at the guard to stop getting me all agitated. Then they write me up another 115 [a disciplinary ticket] for disrespecting an officer and I have to do more time in this rotten hole!"

## What Kind of Treatment Do They Receive?

In prison, security concerns take priority over clinical concerns. Since danger is omnipresent, the security staff retain authority over every aspect of correctional care. This can mean deep trouble for mentally disordered prisoners. For instance, in many high-security prisons, when violence erupts on the yard, the armed guards in the towers or on top of the buildings yell "Down!" and all prisoners are required to fall to the ground, face down. The guards shoot the prisoners who fail to get down. Many prisoners taking psychotropic medications are unable to react to the command in time because their reactions are slowed, either by their illness or by the medications. I have read several reports of prisoners who were taking antipsychotic medications being shot and even killed in this manner. And I have heard from quite a few mentally ill prisoners that they voluntarily remain in their cells all day because they are afraid of being shot in this fashion if they go to the yard. But the guards cite security on the yard as the reason for the shootings, and mentally ill prisoners are left to suffer the consequences.

If a mentally disordered prisoner gets into a fight, it is the security officers and not the mental health staff who intervene. And the consequence is punishment, not an intensification of mental health treatment. In fact, if a prisoner is housed on a special tier designated for a mental health treatment program, and the prisoner-patient gets into a fight with another prisoner-patient or disrespects a security officer on the unit, he or she will be transferred to a punitive detention section of the prison and will no longer be eligible for the treatment program. If the psychiatrist who was treating him complains about staff losing sight of clinical issues in the rush to punish, that psychiatrist will lose credibility with the security staff and consequently find it much more difficult to do his or her job.

Correctional psychiatrists who sincerely care about their patients tell me they often feel that the security staff intervene too quickly and too forcefully with their patients, and fail to consult with the mental health team before doing so. Of course, there are many times when mental health clinicians need the security staff to intervene, if only to ensure the clinician's safety. But at other times, just when they are beginning to gain the trust of a previously recalcitrant prisoner who had been refusing to take his medications, the security staff discipline the disturbed prisoner for a relatively minor offense and the angry prisoner henceforth refuses psychiatric treatment. There are many other variations on the theme.

## Deadly Assistance

The way security staff handle a problem involving a mentally disordered prisoner can be quite counter-therapeutic, even deadly. For instance:

> Steven, a man suffering from severe and long-standing mental illness, was taken to jail on July 25, 1995 because of "outstanding warrants." He was not unlike a large number of mental patients today: dually diagnosed (mental illness plus substance abuse), taking lithium, and living in a board and care home. He told the intake social worker that he was being treated at the county outpatient mental health facility, and that when he gets anxious he tends to slap his face. The social worker ordered the man taken to a safety cell in the eighth floor psychiatric unit.
>
> Steven was not violent, was cooperating fully, and had not even begun to slap himself when five large officers took hold of his limbs, forced him to a supine position on the floor, placed him in a double hammer lock and exerted enough pressure upwards on his two arms and twisted both his wrists forcefully enough to cause him to cry out

in pain. While two officers pressed their knees on the back of his chest, he bit himself, began to spit blood and was clearly having trouble breathing. The officers "blanketed" him, that is, they threw a blanket around his head and twisted it at the neck. He was stripped naked. Then, with two officers holding his arms and two more lifting his legs, he was carried, face down, to the elevator. (This procedure is termed "suitcasing.") One of the officers also pulled up on the blanket. Steven was screaming in pain.

When they arrived on the eighth floor psychiatric unit they roughly threw him down on the safety cell bed. At this point Steven stopped breathing, but this fact went unnoticed for four minutes while jail staff busied themselves applying four-point restraints (tying all four limbs to the bed). When an officer finally noticed that Steven had stopped breathing, there was an ineffectual attempt at CPR. Steven never emerged from the coma.

When security staff view every situation from a security perspective, terrible things happen to mentally ill prisoners. When the staff assume that every prisoner who asks for psychiatric attention is merely manipulating to get into a more comfortable setting (I explore this issue in Chapter Three), mentally disordered prisoners' problems are compounded. And when the security staff insist that a mentally disordered prisoner who has been assaulted must disclose the identity of the perpetrator before they will permit him or her to receive help, they are creating unbearable stress on the already disabled prisoner. In other words, security staff can be very unsympathetic toward the prisoners they control, especially toward those suffering from mental disorders. And a lack of sympathy can cause great harm.

## Two Routes to Solitary

As I tour prisons I am alarmed by the number of prisoners who remain in their cells with the lights out in the middle of the day, and by the number of severely disturbed prisoners I find in lock-up units of all kinds, especially the supermaximum security units. Neither situation is conducive to healing broken psyches. Yet a large number of mentally disordered prisoners, lacking a setting where they feel safe enough to come out of their cells, opt to remain cell-bound. At the same time, another large group may go to the day-rooms and yard, get into trouble, and get punished by being sent to "the hole." There are very dire consequences to both options.

## Self-Induced Cell-Confinement

Many mentally disordered prisoners choose to stay in their cells all day to avoid trouble. Isolation tends to worsen depressions. One African-American man in a high-security general population cell-block confided to me that he is suffering from a severe depression, but still he chooses to stay in his cell all day and never go out on the yard. He tells me he sleeps more than fourteen hours per day, but is afraid to seek psychiatric attention: "Even if I could get an appointment with a shrink, he'd only see me for a few minutes and put me on some kind of pills. I don't want anyone messing with my mind, giving me pills that keep me from thinking straight. I gotta keep my wits about me so I can stay out of trouble and finish out my term. I'm short [nearing the end of his sentence]. I'd rather be depressed and stay by myself than go out on the yard and get into a hassle and have them throw me into lock-up and add time onto my sentence."

The social isolation and sensory deprivation that are part of confinement to a cell worsen psychotic conditions. In many cases, a psychotic prisoner retreats to his cell, and because he is able to survive there and continue to eat the meals he is served there or in the cafeteria, his psychotic condition is never declared disabling and he never receives very aggressive treatment.

While preparing to testify in *Gates* v. *Deukmejian*, a class action lawsuit concerning the quality of mental health care at California's Correctional Medical Facility (CMF), I encountered a man who had been "toplocked" (locked in his cell around the clock and fed all meals in his cell for several months) because he was acting too bizarrely to be released into the dining area or the yard.

I testified about this man in the federal court proceeding in 1989: "He was a man who was clearly psychotic. He was confined to his cell. He was unable to program with the other individuals. The prison psychiatrist said that he was very psychotic; however, he was rejected for admission to the small psychiatric inpatient unit within the prison walls by the assessment team because he was still able to eat—although he was not able to shower." I was asked to describe the man: "I believe he had no shirt on. He was sitting on the floor and mumbling to himself. I didn't do a psychiatric examination. But he had the hair-on-the-back-of-the-neck sign. That is, when you walk up to someone and you can tell, because the hair on the back of your neck stands up, that this individual is psychotic. And he definitely had that sign."

Not all mentally ill prisoners who choose to remain in their cells are as severely disturbed as the prisoner I described in court that day. But no matter how mild or severe their psychiatric symptoms, confinement in a cell with no real social interaction or meaningful activity tends to exacerbate all types of mental disorders.

## Striking Out and Going to the "Hole"

Other prisoners suffering from serious mental disorders, because they are not very good at controlling their impulses, strike out at the least provocation and are sent to lock-up, where the isolation and stressful conditions cause further deterioration of their psychiatric condition. For example:

> James is a forty-three-year-old African-American man serving time in a security housing unit of a state prison system who is unusual among prisoners in having a bachelors degree from a prestigious university. When I met him he was in the eighth year of a fifty-year sentence for murdering his father. He had no prior criminal record, and he swears the death was accidental. "I loved my father very much, it

was just one of those freak accidents. We were arguing, my sister had told him I was ripping off some money he had me managing for the family—that was a lie, he wouldn't believe me—there was a gun he had for protection, I shot him."

James had been struggling to control his temper outbursts all of his life, and had done relatively well until his father's death. Once he entered prison he began getting into fights and arguing with the guards. He received many disciplinary write-ups, and eventually was sent to the Security Housing Unit. He says he wants to take an anger management course, but he has never been given the opportunity.

James was hesitant to answer my questions about suicide, but tears appeared when I raised the subject. He began the interview with a studied composure, but as we continued to talk his thoughts became more disorganized. He eventually admitted he heard voices, and believed someone was trying to use him to channel thoughts from another world. He reported a beating that had occurred a few months earlier while he was being transported in shackles—the officer who was accompanying him pulled up on the "leash" (a strap connected to the handcuffs, wrapped under the leg irons and held by a guard who walks behind the prisoner) throwing him face first into the concrete floor. Then two guards pounced on him and kicked and beat him. I asked why they would do that, and he admitted he doesn't really know, "But maybe it has something to do with the fact that I'm one of a very small number of prisoners—or guards for that matter—who have been through college, so maybe they feel like I'm trying to down them."

As the interview continued he let down his guard and shared with me some of the ideas that he usually keeps to himself: He has immense sexual powers on account of an undescended testicle that remains lodged in his abdomen, and that is the real reason most men feel immense envy in his presence and want to attack him. He only gets into fights to protect himself from their assaults. In fact, "I keep hearing voices telling me that this prisoner or that guard is about to jump me, so I have to make the first move." But then his more rational side takes over and he tells me the fighting gets him locked up in solitary, where he obsesses about killing his father, cries a lot, and thinks constantly about killing himself. James is far from the most severely disturbed felon I have found in a supermaximum control unit, but clearly the harsh environment blocks his attempts to learn to control his temper, and his situation is not at all conducive to effective mental health treatment.

Often it is the symptoms of the mental disorder that cause the prisoner to be sent to a lock-up unit.

Sam is African American, muscular, in his mid-twenties. I found him in an administrative segregation unit in a state prison, where he had been placed after a fight with a cellmate. He reports experiencing flashbacks to the crime that brought him to prison. In fact, the fight with his cellmate began when he looked at his "cellie's" face and saw the bloody face of the man his crime-partner had murdered. He was frightened, but because he had learned to turn fear into rage in order to survive in prison, he attacked his cellmate.

Sam had no psychiatric record, and no criminal record, prior to being arrested for doing "a job" with a buddy. He thought it was a simple burglary: They would enter a store, take something, and run. They were caught in the act. A store security guard ran after them. His friend pulled a gun, turned, and fired. The bullet hit the guard in the face and the man fell dead. To this day he cannot get the image of the guard's face out of his mind. In fact, he is often wakened by nightmares in which the guard's bloody face appears to torment him. He suffers from severe, chronic insomnia and tells me he is unable to concentrate, even enough to read a book. He also startles very easily, in reaction to a sudden noise or someone entering a room unexpectedly. And he answers affirmatively to most of the items on a symptom checklist for posttraumatic stress disorder.

Sam tends to isolate himself, but periodically someone bumps into him or takes something he thinks belongs to him and he explodes with rage. He shows me some of the wounds he has accumulated, including a scar across his abdomen, "from the time surgeons had to remove my spleen after a fight." There is another scar on his shoulder where he was stabbed, a scar at the point of entry of a bullet and another at the point of exit. He tells me that he never got into fights before entering prison. As a child, he did witness his drunken father beat his mother many times, and he was only ten when he first saw a "drive-by" where someone died. Since entering prison, he has been involved in many fights. He explains that is why he spends so much time in lock-up.

## A Very Vicious Cycle

Erving Goffman, Thomas Scheff, and other "sociologists of deviance" described a vicious cycle that was at play in the age of "snakepit" mental asylums. A man is identified as disturbed, and on account of that designation his freedom is constricted and he is denied certain means of self-expression. Perhaps he is locked on a ward without company, telephone, or meaningful activity. He acts out, for instance, by throwing a chair through a window in order to express as best he can his dissatisfaction with the deprivation. Then he is locked in even tighter security, for instance a smaller room without windows or furniture, while the staff conclude that his chair-throwing proves he was disturbed enough to warrant the kind of deprivations they had earlier forced on him, and congratulate themselves for having correctly assessed the severity of his problem in the first place. Then the man is left in the isolation room with no other way to express himself, so he does something even more bizarre, such as smear feces on the walls. And again his subsequent actions convince his keepers they were wise to throw him into the isolation room.

Obviously this formulation fits the career of psychotic prisoners who wind up in supermaximum control units. A SHU is the most intensive form of lock-up, but not the only one. Most medium and high-security prisons contain some kind of lock-up capacity. Except when they are housed in dormitories, all prisoners can be toplocked. Often prisoners who are considered suicidal or acutely psychotic are toplocked until the staff can figure out whether to transfer them to a psychiatric unit. And any prison can be "locked down," meaning that all prisoners are locked in their cells or dorms, a measure that is usually instituted following an outbreak of violence. Additionally, most prisons contain an Ad Seg unit. Some of the prisoners housed in Ad Seg are being punished for disciplinary infractions, some are mentally disturbed or suicidal, some are in need of protective custody, and some are there because the administration cannot figure out anything else to do with them. Medium- and high-security prisons usually contain a punitive segregation unit as well, sometimes called a Security Housing Unit or SHU, where most of the prisoners serving lock-up terms for disciplinary infractions are housed.

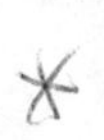

With mentally ill prisoners, the staff usually decide that although this prisoner may be suffering from a mental disorder, his or her recalcitrance and violent outbursts reflect "badness" rather than "madness," and this is why punishment is instituted and not treatment. But even the notion of badness requires careful scrutiny. It is very true that many prisoners housed in control units have committed very deplorable acts, including the original crime for which they were sentenced and violent acts during their prison term. (These units are also utilized to isolate jailhouse lawyers, political leaders, and others who are deemed by wardens to constitute security risks in prisons.) But if we leave it at that, as though any kind of cruel punishment is their due for past crimes, then we are very likely to cause them to become more violent and depraved in the future because of the traumas they suffer while in lock-up.

I do not in any way mean to imply that prisoners who commit illegal or violent acts should not be punished. But the mass warehousing of a large number of rule-breaking prisoners in lock-up units increases the likelihood that these men and women will resort to worse violence and antisocial acts in the future—during their terms of incarceration or after their release.

This vicious cycle applies to psychotic as well as nonpsychotic prisoners. I have seen or heard of quite a few cases of feces-slinging in the supermax security units I have toured, and the prisoners involved in the slinging are not always overtly psychotic. Some explain they are "bombing" or "gassing" the guards because it is the only form of retaliation they can muster in response to what they consider brutal and unfair treatment. Others tell me that they have thrown excrement at another prisoner, often a mentally disordered one, only in retaliation for an earlier equivalent barrage. Sometimes it is not possible to determine precisely which prisoners in such a setting are severely disturbed. Some have learned to hide their symptoms, others are too paranoid to permit a clinician to examine them, and, yes, some are faking their symptoms—but not as many as the guards and mental health staff accuse.

Felons as a group are not known for their capacity to control anger or follow orders. Several ex-felons I treat in my office tell me that their best chance of avoiding trouble is to walk away from it. They have learned, after many brushes with the law, to seek a silent exit whenever they are provoked and angered. But in prison there is no exit. A forty-three-year-old African-American prisoner in a supermax unit explained to me why he gets into fights and has to be sent to lock-up: "You have angry thoughts. They won't leave your mind. You want to get back at someone who's hurt you. On the outside, you can walk away and find your composure. Here you can't walk away or hide. Once someone gets to you, they keep going at you—C.O.'s [correctional officers] and other inmates—they'll say you snitched or something." Prisoners are routinely challenged by other prisoners to fight, or they find themselves in authority conflicts with staff. As a general rule, each time they are written up and sent to a more restrictive level of custody, the new setting permits less deviance and less opportunity to exit a potentially explosive situation silently—there is nowhere to go. When a prisoner in a lock-up unit answers a guard's question sarcastically, or does not respond quickly enough to a direct order, he is written up anew, or the guard decides to taunt him or use physical force to make him comply.

At the Special Management Unit at Pennsylvania's State Correctional Institution (SCI) at Greene, prisoners are required to progress through five phases of programming, from Phase V, where inmates are deprived of all amenities, to Phase I, where they are permitted more visits and slightly more freedom of movement during "yard time." It takes at least three months to complete each phase, so once a prisoner lands in this unit it takes at least fifteen months to be returned to the general population. An inmate who "maxed out" of this control unit (his prison term ended prior to the end of his time in the SMU, so the correctional system was required to release him directly to the community) informed me that often an inmate works his way to the end of phase two, or even into phase one, and then a guard "hassles him and he is so irritable by this time from being locked up for so long that he gives him lip." The prisoner's punishment is a return to the beginning of the progression, phase V, and he has to progress through all the phases anew. Since confinement in this kind of isolation unit tends to increase irritability and provoke violent outbursts, it is extremely difficult for a prisoner to traverse all of the five phases successfully and be released from this control unit. My informant continues:

> Some guys do get out, but when they get back to general population they are put on a very tight probation. For instance, there is a rule against walking on certain areas of grass on the population yard, but usually the guards don't really hassle you for walking on the grass. But if you're on probation from lock-up, they write you up the second you stray onto that patch of grass. Then it's back to the SMU and begin those five phases all over again. I've seen a lot of guys crack under the pressure, they go stark-raving mad.

At each step along the way from general population to the isolation unit and cell extractions, the correctional staff think their earlier assumptions about just how bad these prisoners really are have been born out by this new example of recalcitrance and disrespect for authority. Meanwhile, the prisoner is more convinced he is being disrespected and abused, he becomes even angrier, and he is even less willing or able to follow the incrementally stricter rules.

---

I end this chapter with a case that illustrates the built-in vicious cycle at play in prisons today.

Earl is a thirty-three-year-old Caucasian man who has been in the Security Housing Unit of a state prison system for almost three years. He did very poorly in school (he believes he had a learning disability related to childhood fevers and seizures), and even with special education classes he was unable to complete junior high school. His psychiatric history dates to early childhood, as does a severe seizure disorder. His father, a Korean War veteran, was disabled, alcoholic, and abusive. His mother supported the family by working as a nursing assistant.

Earl grew up in a low-income neighborhood where "all the kids committed petty thefts, but they got away with it and I was always the one who got caught—I think I was just too disturbed to plan a getaway or to think up a good alibi." He has been diagnosed and is being treated for a "manic-depressive disorder with psychotic features," but he also suffers from a severe anxiety disorder with panic attacks and intense phobia connected with being confined in a cell.

Earl dates the origin of his "cell phobia" to the time he first arrived in prison ten years earlier and was dragged into a cell and raped repeatedly by several other prisoners. Indeed, besides a history of severe mood swings and psychotic episodes, he exhibits many of the features of chronic posttraumatic stress disorder, including flashbacks, severe insomnia dating back to the rape, nightmares, an intense startle reaction, a greatly constricted life and, of course, the panic attacks. He was written up for his first disciplinary infraction in prison because he refused to follow a direct order by a correctional officer to reenter his cell. He explains that at the moment he refused the order he was more afraid of being confined in the cell then he was concerned about certain punishment for disobeying an order. But his punishment was more confinement in his cell.

Earl also mutilates himself by cutting. I ask him why he cuts and he describes very poignantly how, after he has been confined to a cell for awhile, his anxiety level rises to an unbearable degree and he feels compelled to cut himself. He thinks the cutting is the only way to alleviate the anxiety. Eventually he discovered that each time he cut himself, across the wrist or across the abdomen, he would be removed from his cell and sent to the infirmary for stitches.

"Once I get to the infirmary I calm down immediately, the panic disappears as soon as I get out of that cell." But since self-mutilation is a violation of prison rules, more time is added to his term in lock-up. When I point out that he is taken to the infirmary only for a short time for emergency treatment and then he is returned to his cell, Earl responds: "Still, it's worth it!" He believes the panic he feels in the cell leaves him no other option, and he feels that even the short period of relief is worth the pain and trauma.

Earl, like many of the emotionally disturbed prisoners I find in lock-up units, is entirely dysfunctional, even in the context of the SHU. Most of the time he is too anxious to pursue any line of thought or to read or write, so he paces or lies in bed restlessly during the days and most of the nights, attempting to track his racing thoughts. He is terrified of being confined in a cell, yet he is confined in one nearly twenty-four hours per day. And this vicious cycle only serves to perpetuate and intensify the anxiety and self-mutilation. Earl is one of a large group of very disturbed prisoners who are being punished instead of being treated for their psychiatric disorders.

Of course, the rationale for instituting harsh security precautions and stark deprivations in prison is to prevent violence. But is violence prevented, or bred? Is mental illness contained, or exacerbated? For many reasons, including the defunding of public mental health programs in the community and the inadequacies of mental health services inside, prisons have become warehouses for a huge number of severely disturbed people. When prisoners are denied satisfaction of basic human needs—such as adequate contact with loved ones, a decent private space to live in, some modicum of control over the environment, some say about their privileges and deprivations, some productive outlet and a chance to learn and grow—they become increasingly resentful. Fear, hostility, and confusion well up inside them. Some act violently, in impotent acts like disobeying an order, throwing garbage, or yelling at an officer.

As one inmate stated: "The only way to get anyone to listen to you around here is to totally bug out or hurt someone!" Others break down, or try to kill themselves. But in most prisons self-injury is against the rules, so time is added to their lock-up sentence. A population of hateful prisoners is bred who have few options to express self, who are made incapable of being intimate and tender, and who are not prepared to work or live outside the prison setting.

Though a very large number of prisoners suffer from serious mental disorders, they do not receive adequate treatment. Instead, they are brutalized by staff and prisoners alike. A large subgroup of mentally disordered felons entered prison with histories of serious mental illness, but another large subgroup developed the disturbances that make their lives miserable only after being incarcerated. In Chapter Two I explore some of the stressors that cause so many prisoners to suffer emotional breakdowns in prison.

2

# Why So Many Prisoners Develop Mental Disorders

More offenders with a history of mental illness are being sent to correctional facilities. In addition, harsh prison conditions cause even more prisoners to suffer breakdowns or commit suicide, and inadequate diagnosis and treatment of mental illness behind bars lead to more severe and chronic cases. Predisposing factors for mental illness include massive early childhood trauma, and prisoners as a group report an inordinate amount of severe trauma in their pasts. A significant number of prisoners display the classic signs and symptoms of posttraumatic stress disorder, while another large group of prisoners react to trauma by developing other kinds of psychiatric disturbance. Prison overcrowding increases the violence and makes life inside miserable for everyone, but especially for prisoners with traumatic pasts who are suffering from (or prone to) posttraumatic stress disorder (PTSD) and other serious mental illnesses.

From all the tours and interviews I have conducted, a composite picture stands out of a mentally disordered prisoner: He or she suffered massive and repeated traumas early in life, had great difficulty coping with the stress of harsh prison conditions, and then acted out and was sent to a punitive segregation unit where the isolation and idleness aggravated the mental disorder. This composite reflects the plight of a large number of prisoners who find themselves caught in a downward spiral into madness and despair.

## Traumatic Lives

We are learning that the lives of low-income, inner-city children are filled with trauma. We know that early trauma plays a part in the etiology of all kinds of mental disorders, including posttraumatic stress disorder, psychosis, and severe depression. Since an overwhelming majority of prisoners hail from the inner cities, we should not be surprised to find that their backgrounds include many traumatic occurrences. Unfortunately, their prison careers are full of massive trauma as well. In fact, the daily traumas of prison life can serve, psychologically speaking, as reenactments of the earlier traumas, and the combination of old and new traumas can have a devastating effect on prisoners' mental health.

Posttraumatic stress disorder is usually underdiagnosed in prison. Correctional staff are too little concerned about the part that early trauma plays in the etiology of all forms of serious mental disorders, and they are almost oblivious to the danger, in terms of prisoners' eventual prognoses and potential for postrelease adjustment, of the reenactment of trauma in prison.

### Childhood Trauma

Inner-city children experience or witness an extraordinary amount of trauma. By the time they reach high school, 35 percent of inner city, African-American children have witnessed a stabbing, 39 percent have personally viewed a shooting, almost 25 percent have seen someone murdered, and 46 percent have been the victim of at least one violent crime. Low-income children of all races experience a shocking amount of domestic violence as the victims of physical and emotional abuse or as witnesses to spousal abuse. We are also learning about a significant amount of sexual abuse among children living in poverty. Poverty itself is traumatic, if not violent.

Whether as victims or witnesses, boys who experience violence and other traumas connected with life in the inner city tend to react in one of two ways: They withdraw into isolation or they become enraged, strike out, and get into trouble. Whereas boys are more likely to exhibit "conduct disorders," traumatized girls tend to become depressed or anxious. Many children who have suffered repeated traumas are rendered incapable of paying attention in class and applying themselves to their schoolwork, so they tend to fail in school. More often than counterparts who do well in school, some of these children drift into criminal paths, often drug-related, and a certain number eventually get caught. Given diminishing resources in public education and public mental health services, inner-city youths who act out aggressively are more likely to be punished than to be treated. In other words, childhood trauma is one of the mechanisms that cause the underclasses and people of color to be vastly overrepresented in our jails and prisons.

A large majority of prisoners come from low-income, high-crime neighborhoods, and report repeated and prolonged trauma and violence since childhood. A significant proportion of sexually assaultive adolescent males were themselves victims of sexual abuse as children. Sixty-eight percent of youth offenders in Oregon treatment programs were abused as children or witnessed their mothers being abused. The proportion of offenders with histories of childhood physical abuse is much higher, and family violence has been shown to be pervasive in the histories of violent adolescents. Men who witnessed violence between their parents are three times more likely to commit domestic violence than those who grew up in less abusive homes. A recent Massachusetts study found that children from violent homes are twice as likely as nontraumatized children to commit violent crimes, six times more likely to commit suicide, and twenty-four times as likely to be the perpetrators of sexual assault. And over 40 percent of incarcerated women suffered physical or sexual abuse prior to their arrest.

Almost every prisoner on death row reports a childhood filled with severe trauma. Their stories surface in presentencing reports and psychiatric examinations conducted during the appeals process. I have read many reports and written several myself. Typically, there were alcoholic parents, spousal abuse between the parents, physical and sexual abuse of the child, street violence, and so forth. Every one of the men I have interviewed who were convicted of murder and sentenced to a life sentence or death express intense rage about the way they were treated all of their lives.

Of course, not all individuals who grow up in high-crime neighborhoods develop symptoms of PTSD or other serious mental disorders, nor do all embark on a life of crime. But even though a large number of inner-city youths avoid psychiatric disability and the criminal justice system altogether, it remains the case that a disproportionate number get into serious trouble. I do not mean to imply that it is the psychopathology of the criminals that singularly accounts for crime. Pervasive poverty, racism, poor schools, and high unemployment also play their parts in the social tragedy. Still, evidence is accumulating for a link between the high degree of trauma experienced by children in the inner city and the high incidence of criminal behavior among men and women who grew up there.

## Prisoners with PTSD

Trauma plays a very big part in the lives of potential felons, but when they eventually land in prison the trauma in their backgrounds goes relatively unnoticed. If they develop the signs and symptoms of posttraumatic stress disorder, they are systematically undertreated because correctional mental health services are simply inadequate. We know that left untreated, and especially if the traumatized individual is isolated and unable to work through the ensuing emotional reactions, PTSD worsens.

This is not to say PTSD should be a reason to declare a criminal defendant not guilty by reason of insanity, or even to establish diminished capacity. That issue is being debated, and I will not discuss it here. But whether or not society wishes to consider the criminal's history of trauma in assigning sentences, we definitely need to think long and hard about subjecting previously traumatized convicts to severe and unnecessary retraumatization during their stays in correctional facilities.

> Ron is a forty-seven-year-old African-American man who is serving a term of over a century for the only crime for which he was ever convicted: He killed his wife and children. After returning from combat duty in Vietnam he married, worked in a factory, and lived with his wife and children. The company he worked for moved its operations overseas to reduce labor costs, the domestic factory was closed, and Ron lost his job. One night he consumed a large amount of alcohol, and an argument erupted between him and his wife. She screamed at him, he marched upstairs to get his gun and returned to shoot her and the children. That was over twenty years ago. Today he is sitting in a prison cell, ruminating obsessively about his crime.
>
> Ron is pleasant and articulate. The high-security prison is usually reserved for those with known gang-affiliations or disciplinary problems, but he was assigned there because of his long sentence. He told me that he spends almost all of his time in his cell thinking about his wife and kids. He is clearly depressed and there are signs of delusions. He complains of nightmares that keep him up most nights. He says he experiences flashbacks, often feels numb, suffers panic attacks, and is very irritable and jumpy. He cannot concentrate even though he tries to get his mind off his family by reading everything he can get his hands on. And he feels totally isolated from the other inmates. Two psychiatrists testified during his trial that he was clearly psychotic at the time he murdered his family. There is one note in his prison chart that mentions the possibility he might be suffering from PTSD along with a recurring psychotic condition. Yet very little treatment has been offered him in prison. He feels that he needs someone to talk to, "Or else I'm going to explode! Or commit suicide!"

There are many reasons that PTSD is underdiagnosed and undertreated in prisons. One technical reason for the underdiagnosis of

PTSD is the *either/or* assumption of clinicians. Much of clinical research is based on the assumption that a prisoner is *either* suffering from one disorder *or* another, but not both. Thus, if a prisoner exhibits the signs and symptoms of psychosis, that diagnostic label is applied and the search for psychopathology ceases. But it is very possible for a person to suffer from both psychosis and posttraumatic stress disorder—as in Ron's case—and it is quite possible for a psychotic episode to be set off by a traumatic incident. In fact, a large number of cases of PTSD among prisoners are being missed because so many eventually decompensate into psychosis and then clinicians miss the connection between the current psychiatric symptomatology and the traumas, past and present.

There are also structural reasons for the underdiagnosis of PTSD in prison. For instance, in an institution where resources for mental health services are scarce, only the most severely disturbed and acutely suicidal patients receive clinical attention. The mental health staff are instructed to ignore minor forms of madness and concentrate on "major mental illnesses" such as schizophrenia and major affective disorders, and cases that present an immediate serious risk of suicide. Even though posttraumatic stress disorder, panic disorder, social phobia, and other "nonmajor" forms of mental illness can cause significant suffering and disability, the overextended mental health staff tend to ignore them. It is as if they figure, "Why diagnose what we do not have the resources to treat?"

## Two Reactions to Trauma

The images of two groups of prisoners stand out in my mind: the large number of men and women who remain in their bunks with the lights out in the middle of the day; and the large number of prisoners who are locked in some form of segregated, security housing units. When I talk to prisoners who choose to remain in their cells most of the time, I am told it is not safe to go on the yard, that they want to stay to themselves so they can do their time without getting into trouble. But this is precisely the kind of social and emotional constriction that typically follows extreme trauma. Many of these men and women are depressed and experience some of the intrusive and constrictive symptoms of PTSD. Some are suicidal. But the self-imposed isolation makes sense, given the dangerous situation prisoners find themselves in and the lack of quality treatment options.

Meanwhile, another group of men and women exhibit a different coping style. When they are disrespected or treated badly, they strike out verbally and physically toward offending cons and guards. They tend to get "locked up." One might say these men and women carry a chip on their shoulder. They say that the guards are constantly harassing them, conducting unnecessary cell-searches, making trouble, provoking violence, and so forth. It seems likely that a significant proportion of these prisoners, if they were in a less stressful place, would not go over the edge quite so often. But take a group of men and women with traumatic pasts and quick tempers and place them in a frightening situation such as the yard of an overcrowded prison, and a significant number will end up in a fight or talk back to a correctional officer and get thrown in "the hole."

Rule-breaking can be a sign of PTSD. But prison staff do not view rule-breaking as a sign of mental illness and they are much more likely to order punishment than treatment. Once labeled troublemakers, these prisoners tend to get into more trouble. Part of the problem is the "rep" they have to maintain. Part is the tendency for guards to look to known troublemakers as the culprits whenever new trouble erupts. But lock-down is about the worst treatment one could design for someone suffering from PTSD. And then that old self-fulfilling prophecy is put in play: The lock-down makes traumatized prisoners ever more irritable and rageful, and the guards point to the growing rage as proof they were right to lock them down.

It has been my impression during the course of my tours that a significant number of the men and women who stay in their cells with the lights out all day, and a large number of those sequestered in disciplinary segregation, exhibit the signs and symptoms of PTSD and other trauma-induced mental disorders. Remember, children who are traumatized tend to react in two ways, by striking out and getting into trouble or by withdrawing into defeatism and depression. It seems the childhood patterns continue for a lifetime. In the course of interviewing several hundred prison inmates, I have discovered a significant number of men and women who exhibit some or all of the essential features of PTSD.

## Trauma and Severe Mental Disorders

Responses to stress take many forms. The classic case of PTSD involves flashbacks, nightmares, panic attacks, aggravated startle reactions, hypervigilance, numbing, and other forms of emotional constriction. But if a person who is prone to suffer "major" forms of emotional breakdown undergoes a severe trauma, the event can precipitate a psychotic or depressive breakdown instead of the classic syndrome known as PTSD. The intrusive images are woven into the hallucinations and delusions, and we miss the connection between the trauma and the breakdown. For example:

> Robert spent some time in a state mental hospital prior to his arrest and conviction. He seemed to be of sound mental health during his processing through the prison reception center. Then he was gang-raped. He did not report the assault for fear of retaliation, but he soon began to experience hallucinations and delusions. When the psychotic symptoms became obvious and the guards finally noticed his condition, he was sent to see a psychiatrist, who prescribed anti-psychotic medications.

Ignoring the effects of trauma in prisoners runs certain risks. The risk to the prisoners is that the repeated traumas they are forced to endure during incarceration worsen their psychiatric conditions and their prognoses. There are also grave social consequences. After all, most of these convicts do eventually go free, and we know from our experience with Viet Nam veterans suffering from PTSD that there can be chronic depression and disability as well as many cases of suicide. And then there are those unpredictable and seemingly inexplicable violent outbursts. Prisoners who have suffered severe and repeated traumas in the past are prone to suffer from debilitating emotional reactions when they are retraumatized. Since harsh prison conditions and solitary confinement constitute pretty severe traumas for most prisoners, this toxic combination of past and present trauma is one big reason so many prisoners suffer from serious mental disorders today.

## Crowding and Other Harsh Conditions

With the explosive growth of the prison population since 1980, prison crowding is rampant in most state and federal facilities and getting worse, even with all the prison construction mandated by federal and state anticrime bills. Many prisons are filled to 150 or 200 percent of their design capacity. Double-celling is pervasive. Dorms are crowded well beyond capacity. The typical cell in older prisons is six feet wide and eight feet long, with a sink-and-toilet fixture at the end opposite the cell door, and a single bed stretching from the door nearly to the other end. A large man has to turn sideways to walk along the side of the bed. When there are two cellies and the single bed is replaced by a bunk set-up, one of them has to stay in bed if the other is to walk to the toilet or the door. In addition, many dayrooms and gymnasiums have been converted into makeshift dorms.

There is a growing body of research linking crowding with increases in the prevalence of violence, psychiatric disturbances, and suicide. In 1962 Calhoun demonstrated a link in rats between overcrowding and increased infant mortality, violence, and social disorganization. Since then, researchers have been examining the effects of overcrowding on humans in prisons and other confined spaces. People who are prone to impulsive behavior, rule-breaking, and psychiatric disturbances do not fare well when they are crowded. The crowding constitutes an intolerable trauma in itself. The rise in violence creates many new traumas, especially for the vulnerable, mentally disordered felon.

Prisoners who have a history of psychiatric breakdowns are more likely to suffer relapses, and many other prisoners who have never suffered a significant psychiatric disturbance in the past report worrisome psychiatric symptoms for the first time. Suicide rates rise with the upswing in violence and emotional breakdowns.

## How Crowding Affects Behavior

The effects of prison crowding are obvious to the visitor. In some of the state prisons I have toured, between 100 and 250 prisoners are housed in bunk beds placed close together in a gymnasium the size of a basketball court. There is no privacy in these huge dorms. There are lines to use the toilet and the phone. And there are the inevitable disputes and fights that erupt under such conditions.

Upon entering one of these makeshift dorms, I am struck first by the noise level, including constant shouting, security officers barking orders or calling out inmates' names, and the flushing of the ten or twelve toilets that have been installed along one wall of the gymnasium. The inmates report that the noise never dies down, and there is "always someone hassling you." The lights are usually left on all night, presumably for security reasons, and inmates tell me they have a hard time sleeping. The men bring food to their bunks, so there are roaches and mice. Tempers flare, fights erupt, victimization is rampant.

If inmates are housed in cells, even with a cellmate, they can escape into the cell and lock the door, giving them some respite from the brutality that may be occurring in day areas and yards. But there is no respite for the prisoner who is forced to live in a crowded dorm. There are too many inmates for security staff to supervise adequately. As I entered a very small, crowded, twelve-man dorm where one has to turn sideways to squeeze by the beds, a prisoner explained: "It used to be there were only four beds in this space. There was empty floor space, and a guard walking by could check the whole area. Now, with twelve bunks crowded in here the guard can't see nothin' from the hallway and the guys could be raping someone in one of the back bunks and there'd be no one to stop 'em."

The stress intensifies the tendency for stronger inmates to victimize weaker ones. When a crowded gym dorm is the site of a reception center, where newly admitted felons are housed until they can be classified and assigned a cellblock, there is no cell for a frightened "fish" (newcomer) to hide in, and if he is unable to defend himself against tougher inmates he is at risk for a beating, rape, or worse. And once an inmate is branded a weakling, there will be repeated assaults.

With increased crowding, prisoners are transferred more often from institution to institution according to the availability of empty beds. The prisoners in each facility have shorter track records, on average, so there are fewer unquestioned leaders among the tough guys and more turf battles. The predator has to fight more, perhaps rape more, merely to stay alive. This is one reason the violence level rises. Prisoners with histories of mental illness and prisoners who are prone to decompensate or attempt suicide under extreme duress have an especially difficult time coping with crowded conditions. One subgroup is victimized, another subgroup has trouble controlling their aggressive impulses, and still another subgroup retreats into their cells in an attempt to stay out of trouble.

Of course, there are comparable effects on staff, who must dwell for entire shifts in the same crowded spaces. With greater crowding, the staff is rotated to different assignments and shifts more often, the prisoners are transferred more frequently to other units, and the result is prisoners and staff who know each other less well and have less basis for trust. The larger number of inmates in each area increases the risks for guards, who have to patrol among the inmates without a weapon (so that prisoners cannot attack a guard and procure a dangerous weapon).

Correctional officers freely admit that an overcrowded facility is more dangerous and the work more difficult compared with a prison with a smaller, more familiar, and manageable population. The more anxious correctional officers are about their security, the more likely they are to react defensively and violently when encountering inmates' resistance or taunts. Many staff report they feel burned out from working in large, overcrowded facilities. Others admit that the stress tends to make them take their frustrations out on the prisoners. They are less willing and less able to pay attention to prisoners' complaints about emotional problems, and more likely to respond to rule-breaking on the part of mentally ill prisoners by writing disciplinary "tickets."

Crowding creates many other causes for aggravation. For instance, the wait to see a doctor or a dentist is lengthened. Visiting is more limited in an overcrowded facility, if only because there are limited spots in the visiting areas and the overworked staff are unable to process the visits as rapidly. The food is prepared with less care because the kitchen crew has more prisoners to serve. In addition, since the stress leads to more fights, and most fights end in some kind of disciplinary proceeding, more prisoners are sent to "the hole" or some form of security or isolation housing. The whole prison is more rife with outbursts.

## Other Harsh Conditions

With crowding comes a greater lack of privacy. A lack of privacy is inherent to a certain degree in a prison for security reasons. However, the routine invasions of privacy eventually go far beyond what is necessary and become quite traumatic for the prisoners. There are the repeated, unannounced cell searches, which tend to occur more often when security staff feel threatened by being outnumbered in large, crowded institutions. Body searches regularly include the order to strip. Body cavities are probed. All toilet functions are open to view. Prisoners suffering from paranoia, as well as those who are prone to shaming, have a difficult time coping with the routine.

Crowding is also accompanied by a heightened noise level, worse sanitation, and idleness. Noise itself can traumatize people. Experiments show that people subjected to higher noise levels (from nearby freeways or construction sites, as well as the noise of a prison block) display higher incidences of anxiety and other emotional symptoms. Generally we have some control over the level of noise to which we are subjected. For instance, we can close a door or move into another room to avoid someone playing the stereo, or to the back of the house if there is construction on the street. But in prison the convict has little control over his or her movements, and little or no control over the noise level. The individual prisoner's inability to modify the noise level confronts her once again with her powerlessness and vulnerability, and this helps explain an increased incidence of depression and other mental disorders in crowded facilities.

Hygiene also deteriorates with overcrowding. Sanitation has been grossly deficient in most of the prisons I have visited. In older prisons, toilets are hooked up in such a way that one inmate's flushed waste can back up into his neighbor's toilet or sink. Hot water is often unavailable for showers, and in one cellblock I observed a garden hose being used in lieu of a nonfunctioning shower—in the middle of winter. In a prison where the cafeteria had been burned down during a riot two years earlier, the gutted shell was still standing and connected to the new cafeteria that was in use. The burned and rotting structure, as well as the rotting walls of the current cafeteria, were a breeding place for roaches and other vermin. Some prison kitchens are relatively sanitary, some are gross and disgusting. When I asked an inmate kitchen worker in a less-than-sanitary prison about grease and residue-laden metal trays I observed in the kitchen, he told me that cafeteria work is very low-paying and alienating, and the prisoners who work there just do not pay much attention to cleanliness or sanitation.

I have observed roaches in almost every prison I have visited, particularly in the segregation units where food is served in the cells, and in the makeshift dormitories. In one high-security unit I observed men lying in darkened cells with roaches crawling over them, and heard them report that it is such a common experience that they do not even bother any longer to brush them away. I observed many inmates set traps and catch dozens of roaches in their cells in a span of one or two days. I have also observed pigeon waste inside prison cellblocks, where broken and unrepaired windows serve as entry ports for birds.

The sanitation problems, combined with poor ventilation and inadequate heating (for example, on five-tiered cell-blocks the top tiers are unbearably hot while the bottom ones are very cold in winter), mean that inmates are repulsed by the ever-present stench of human and animal waste and endangered by a heightened risk of infection and infestation. All of this adds to the traumatic effect of imprisonment. And all of this is difficult for an emotionally upset prisoner to bear.

In prisons where the census is far above the prison's rated capacity, idleness is pervasive. The crowding effect is compounded by the dismantling and downsizing of educational and rehabilitative programs that occurred during the same years as the population explosion. There are too few meaningful jobs to go around. The gyms have been converted into dorms, so the recreation facilities are fewer. The increased violence leads to more and longer lock-downs, and a significant number of prisoners break rules and are sent to solitary confinement—which means they lose their jobs and access to classes, the library, and the main yard. Some states are even removing the weights from prison yards. Of course, with fewer meaningful prison jobs and rehabilitation programs, there is less training and productive activity for the prisoners, more idleness, and less hope of "making it" after release.

Common sense tells us that all prisoners tolerate their time in prison better and are more likely to succeed at "going straight" after release if, during the time they serve, the prison has adequate space, the prisoners are permitted some privacy as well as some control over the noise level, the hygiene is adequate, and a certain number of meaningful programs and activities are available. But with overcrowding, double-celling, lack of control over physical conditions, and enforced idleness, more prisoners feel traumatized, suffer psychiatric breakdowns, and commit suicide. The traumas prisoners experience behind bars serve as reminders or reenactments of the multiple traumas they experienced earlier in their lives. Many mentally disordered prisoners have difficulty staying out of trouble, and a disproportionate number wind up in some form of lock-up.

## Breakdowns in Solitary Confinement

By the mid-1980s, severe prison overcrowding and the discontinuation or downsizing of educational and rehabilitation programs led to a heightened level of violent disturbances and psychiatric breakdowns in American prisons. Instead of attempting to remedy the crowding and idleness, correctional authorities opted to build state-of-the-art "maxi-maxi" or "supermaximum control units" or "SHUs," where prisoners who won't conform or who speak out too vehemently are kept in their cells twenty-three or more hours per day, often for years. Forty-one states and the federal prison system now have supermaximum control units. The forced idleness and isolation in these units cause many previously stable men and women to exhibit signs of serious mental illness. But for people who already suffer from mental disorders, the segregation environment is totally intolerable.

Meanwhile, a significant proportion of prisoners with psychiatric problems are selectively funneled into segregated housing. In other words, they misbehave on account of their mental illness, but since they are not likely to be diagnosed and treated adequately, they are punished with time in "the hole." If they attempt suicide or self-mutilation, they are punished for their illegal attempts to harm themselves with more time in punitive segregation.

## Staying Sane in an Insane Environment

Pelican Bay State Prison (PBSP) sits in the middle of a redwood forest just below California's coastal border with Oregon. Driving through the lush forest one suddenly arrives at a broad clearing, in the center of which is a large, concrete, bunker-like structure, surrounded by several hundred yards of gravel. Guards tell me the gravel is meant to cause an escaping prisoner to make a lot of noise as he runs. The buildings are made of concrete and cinder blocks, including the walls and ceilings, and the few small windows cannot be opened. Wall-hangings are not permitted. The prison was built in the late 1980s to replace high-security units such as the "adjustment center" at San Quentin and the Security Housing Units (SHUs) at Folsom and Soledad prisons.

One of the concrete structures is for the general population. The other structure is the Security Housing Unit, a state-of-the-art high-technology supermaximum security unit consisting of "pods," or sections, each with a number of "ranges" branching out from control booths, like spokes from the hub of a wheel. Security officers sit in the control booths with large windows and video screens that permit them to monitor the ranges (rows of cells) and their occupants, and open and close doors by remote control. There is no natural lighting and the lights are on around the clock. The place looks very clean and efficient.

The prisoners, most of whom are double celled, are released one or two at a time to go to the shower or to the small, closed-in space that is called "the yard." But there is no dirt in the yard, merely more concrete floors and walls; there is no view of the sky, merely an opaque plastic roof; and there is little or no recreational equipment. Correctional officers explain that equipment creates a security risk. The inmates take their meals in their cells and must remain there close to twenty-four hours per day. Many refuse to take advantage of the few hours per week they are permitted to go to the yard, and consequently spend even more time in their cells. The architecture minimizes human contact. The inmates cannot see their neighbors and cannot talk to anyone except their cellmate without shouting. There is little reason for the officers to visit the cells except to deliver food, and consequently the hallway in front of the cell doors is empty most of the time. The view seems eerily colorless in all directions, day and night.

An African-American inmate who has been in the SHU for two years describes his experience:

> Sometimes I feel overwhelmed. I get trepidations, nervous, agitated, I go off the deep end. I don't really hear voices, just get to feeling like I can't breathe, the cell is getting smaller. Panic! It feels closed in, my heart pounds, these symptoms build up over days. It feels like I'm suffocating. The next day, before I know it, I'm punching my cellie. It's the SHU that's making me this nervous. There's nothing like this at other prisons. Here I feel like I'm in a kennel, closed off from life itself. I feel like I live in a coffin, like a tomb [he puts his hand to his heart], there's no signs of life around here. At other prisons I could see some form of life out the window. Here, you don't see none of that. That's had an effect on me over the years since I've been here. This is what causes problems with my cellie—I've never had such problems in my life. This environment makes me antagonistic. It's the feeling of being subhuman—it's strange the way it's built—I've never been in an institution like this before.
>
> Once, on the way to the eye doctor, I went outside. I felt like I was born again—look at this, I'm alive! I came back, it made me feel despondent, a gloomy feeling. At the other prison I felt that even though I was in jail, I was happy to be alive. Here, you don't see nothing, just concrete. You never see the sun. In the pod you can't even see the sun through the skylight from your cell.

> There's no form of life, really. I think it has a psychological effect on people—the way it's built. There's a lot of people going crazy. The VCU [violence control unit, a pod in the Security Housing Unit where a plastic door is added to the outside of the cell door to prevent spitting and throwing, and possibly to silence the inmate within] is full of them. It breaks them. A lot of them just cut loose. A lot of things I ain't never seen in other prisons, like cell fights. I never seen this many because these are angry people. The design here, nothing to focus on but your cellie, so you get into a fight. You don't see the sun. . . . I never saw cell fights like this—people get seriously hurt.

This man is quite perceptive and has a lot of what clinicians term "ego strength," a prerequisite to surviving in an environment as extreme as the SHU at Pelican Bay State Prison. I did not think he was psychotic, though he suffered from a fairly severe panic disorder. Imagine what would happen to an inmate who does not have this man's ego strength and is unable to maintain contact with reality under this degree of stress.

## The SHU Syndrome

Every prisoner placed in an environment as stressful as a supermax unit, whether especially prone to mental breakdown or seemingly very sane, eventually begins to lose touch with reality and exhibit some signs and symptoms of psychiatric decompensation, even if the symptoms do not qualify for a diagnosis of psychosis. An inmate who was recently transferred to the SHU of PBSP wrote to me: "Brother I had started talking to myself and I got scared and laughed out loud, I began to think it was OK to answer myself, or should I just talk?" A majority of the inmates I have interviewed in supermaximum control units talk about their inability to concentrate, their heightened anxiety, their intermittent disorientation and confusion, their experience of unreality, and their tendency to strike out at the nearest person when they reach their "breaking point."

Psychiatrist Stuart Grassian examined a large number of prisoners during their stay in segregated, solitary confinement units and concluded that these units, like the sensory deprivation environments that were studied in the 1960s, tend to induce psychosis. Even inmates who do not become frankly psychotic report a number of psychosis-like symptoms, including massive free-floating anxiety, hyper-responsiveness to external stimuli, perceptual distortions and hallucinations, a feeling of unreality, difficulty with concentration and memory, acute confusional states, the emergence of primitive aggressive fantasies, persecutory ideation, motor excitement, violent destructive or self-mutilatory outbursts, and rapid subsidence of symptoms upon termination of isolation. Grassian named this collection of symptoms "the SHU syndrome."

Women prisoners are not immune to this kind of harsh treatment. The women's High-Security Unit (HSU) in Lexington, Kentucky, was a small, underground isolation unit run by the U.S. Bureau of Prisons for two years. It was shut down in August, 1988 in response to international outcries against human rights abuses at the facility. But the federal government opened a similar unit in Florida, and several states, including California, have opened supermaximum security units for women prisoners. In addition to all the stresses encountered by male prisoners in equivalent circumstances, women housed in supermaximum control units are faced with constant voyeurism and sexual harassment by the mostly male staff. Psychologist Richard Korn observed symptoms very similar to the ones listed by Grassian in nonpsychotic women forced to undergo long-term solitary confinement in the supermax unit at Lexington. His list includes claustrophobia, chronic rage reaction, suppressed low-level to severe depression, onset of hallucinatory symptoms, defensive psychological withdrawal, blunting of affect, loss of appetite, general malaise, exacerbation of preexisting medical problems, visual disturbances, and heart palpitations.

It matters quite a bit whether a prisoner in solitary confinement is literate. A large number of prisoners never finished high school, and 40 percent are functionally illiterate (meaning, for instance, they would be unable to write a letter explaining a billing error). This is twice the national rate of functional illiteracy. Some supermax units permit radios and televisions, but a prisoner has to be able to buy or rent one, and even then it can be removed because of a disciplinary infraction. Imagine spending nearly twenty-four hours per day in a cell without any social interactions, and no radio or television. Many prisoners tell me that reading and writing are their only activity besides exercise. If a prisoner cannot read or write, what is he or she to do? The boredom drives many prisoners to distraction, if not into overt psychosis.

## Unusual Punishment

Once the mentally ill prisoner has fallen into the category of troublemaker and the mental health staff have signed off on the case, terrible abuses are likely to follow. They are sent to the segregated and solitary sections of the prisons, where the prisoners are deprived of almost all means of self-expression. Some of the prisoners yell, get into fights, or throw human waste at each other and at guards. Where there is extremity on the part of one side, there is likely to be extremity on the part of the other. The officers conduct "cell extractions," a brutal procedure for removing recalcitrant prisoners from their cells.

Cell extractions occur in lock-up and supermaximum security, or in the cellblocks where mentally ill prisoners are "toplocked." When an inmate in one of these settings refuses to follow an order or becomes belligerent, five or six helmeted officers with padded limbs and bullet-proof vests barge into the cell behind a lexan (sturdy plastic) shield and pin the recalcitrant prisoner against the wall. Then they handcuff and manacle the prisoner and remove him or her from the cell. Judging from my review of numerous incident reports, the inmate is usually roughed up, sometimes quite badly, in many cases ending up in the hospital with multiple injuries.

I have reviewed hundreds of incident reports of cell extractions from prisons in several states. On the incident report there is a space for the officer to fill in the reason that the extraction team was called. On the reports I have reviewed, the most frequently cited reason is that the inmate refused to follow an order to exit his cell. Almost as frequent is: "Inmate refused to return his food tray." Imagine the scene: The officer says through the cell bars "Come over here and cuff up!" The mentally disordered inmate responds "Like hell I'm going to come over there and have you jump on me!" The officer warns the inmate and then calls the cell extraction team.

The inmate is already locked inside a cell. One wonders what harm there would be in waiting until the prisoner is less oppositional, or calling a psychiatrist to see whether she might be able to talk some sense into the recalcitrant mental patient. Or perhaps the officers might consider requiring that the prisoner return his tray prior to being fed again. It is as though the officers are in a hurry to do cell extractions. On a single night in June 1992, at the SHU of Pelican Bay State Prison in California, there were more than fifty cell extractions!

Often, before an extraction team rushes a prisoner, the prisoner is shot with a taser dart fired from a rifle to which it remains connected by a thin wire. When the dart attaches to the prisoner's body, an electrical charge is sent through it that knocks the prisoner unconscious. Mentally ill prisoners in these settings are among the first to get into yelling and excrement-flinging, and are overrepresented among the prisoners who are shot and extracted.

There have been deaths by "tasering" of prisoners who take psychotropic medications. A side effect of many psychiatric drugs is an alteration of electrical conduction in the heart as well as the lowering of a person's "seizure threshold." Everyone has a seizure threshold, the amount of electrical activity in the brain that it takes to cause a grand mal seizure. Medications like Thorazine, Haldol, and the antidepressants are known to lower that threshold. They can also cause heart arrhythmias. Thus a prisoner who is taking a psychiatric medication is more likely than others to have a seizure after being "tasered," or to suffer irregular heartbeats, and these developments can lead to death, especially if the medical response is not optimal.

There had been several deaths by tasering of inmates taking psychiatric medications just prior to the 1989 court proceedings in *Gates v. Deukmejian*, a class action lawsuit concerning the quality of medical and psychiatric care and the treatment of inmates suffering from AIDS at the California Medical Facility at Vacaville. During the course of my expert testimony in that case I explained the mechanism of death by tasering, and why psychiatric patients were at high risk. The judge ruled that no inmate who is taking psychiatric medications shall be tasered. I thought the matter was closed.

A couple of years after the judge's order I was informed by attorneys for the prisoners that correctional staff were no longer using tasers during cell extractions with psychiatric patients. Instead, they were using riot guns, rifle-like grenade launchers that fire 37 mm rubber cylinders. When these guns are used by police at demonstrations, they are fired into a crowd from a distance of fifty or a hundred feet. But in prison, they are fired at a prisoner, or aimed to hit him after ricocheting off a wall, within the confines of a six foot by eight foot cell. I was asked to appear at a formal hearing to give an opinion about this practice.

At the hearing I explained that shooting an inmate at close range with a riot gun runs the risk of death by physical trauma. For instance, hitting a person on the head, in the eye, or even in the abdomen risks serious head trauma, blindness, or a ruptured spleen, respectively. And this kind of shooting is almost certain to cause emotional damage and worsen a psychiatrically disordered inmate's condition. For instance, a delusional prisoner would probably weave the shooting into his delusional system, feel more paranoid, more rageful, and would consequently be more prone to further decompensation. Even if he calmed down immediately after he was knocked unconscious by the rubber projectile, the intensified rage and refueled paranoia would worsen his psychiatric disorder as well as his prognosis. Even nonparanoid prisoners suffer from the trauma. I reported talking to several prisoners who had been extracted in this manner and were suffering from flashbacks, nightmares, insomnia, and panic attacks. I compared the shootings and cell extractions to the cruel treatment undergone by inmates in the "snakepit" asylums of the late 1940s and early 1950s.

## Mentally Ill Prisoners Crack Under the Strain

Unless there has been a court order specifically barring the practice at a specified facility, a large number of mentally ill prisoners are housed in supermaximum control units. The psychiatrist working in the SHU at Wabash Valley Correctional Institution in Indiana told me that approximately 50 percent of the nearly 300 prisoners in that unit suffered from serious mental disorders. The high proportion is no accident. As I explained in Chapter One, a vicious cycle is in play that channels a large number of disturbed inmates into punitive lock-up and eventually into a supermaximum security setting.

In addition, the conditions that cause SHU syndrome in relatively healthy prisoners cause psychotic breakdowns in prisoners who have histories of serious mental disorders, or in prisoners who never suffered a breakdown in the past but are prone to break down when the stress and trauma become exceptionally severe. Glancing at Grassian's list of symptoms, I am struck by the similarity to textbook descriptions of schizophrenia and other psychotic conditions. Even a prisoner who has a strong enough ego to survive a term in solitary confinement without falling apart is likely to report one or more symptoms of the SHU syndrome. But many prisoners are not capable of maintaining their sanity in such an extreme environment.

During a 1982 tour of the Michigan Intensive Program Center (MIPC) in Marquette, I walked onto a tier of sixteen cells where some of the most uncontrollable prisoners were housed. In this unit, the doors were opened and closed by remote control from the guards' station, but instead of using video screens to monitor the prisoners' activities, the guards patrolled a walkway above the cells and looked in on the prisoners. The effect of the architecture was to minimize contact between guards and prisoners. The strangeness of this particular unit became obvious as soon as we entered the "freeway" running between the cells. All the prisoners had built barricades behind the bars at the front of their cells. As I walked down the tier and spoke to several of its inhabitants, I began to suspect that several of the inmates on this tier were suffering from acute psychoses.

One prisoner was quite agitated and screaming at the top of his lungs about a plot involving the guards, the snitches, and the FBI to deny him his manhood. I spoke to the prisoner in the cell immediately across from the agitated man's cell, asking him why he had built a barricade of cardboard and sheets to cover the front of his cell. He explained that the prisoner who was screaming all the epithets often resorted to lobbing "agent orange" (a cup or bottle filled with a mixture of urine and feces) into any cell that was not barricaded. Because there were several obviously psychotic inmates on this tier, and because the code mandated retaliation in the event of an attack, the lobbing of "agent orange" became a daily routine—even for sane prisoners. Similarly, in all the supermax units I have toured, the smearing and throwing of feces is commonplace, and it is difficult even for the psychiatrist to know which of the feces-slinging prisoners are actually psychotic.

Another characteristic of the SHU syndrome is the resolution of symptoms once a prisoner is removed from the extreme environment. I observed this phenomenon in the course of interviewing a single inmate on two occasions, once in the SHU at Pelican Bay State Prison in January 1992, and again in a much less harsh setting, the California Medical Facility in Vacaville in October 1992. At PBSP he was extremely psychotic and was taking a virtual overdose of antipsychotic medications. This emaciated Caucasian man with long hair and a disheveled appearance was clearly hallucinating during our first interview at the SHU, and could not concentrate or think clearly. Yet he exhibited the kind of slurred speech and physical discomfort that accompany an overdose of strong tranquilizers or mood-regulating antiseizure medications (he was taking both). He told me he ate little for fear he was being poisoned—in other words, he remained delusional in spite of the medications—yet he slept most of the day because of the medications' side effects. Still, he seemed to me quite agitated, with a penetrating gaze that I have seen only in very severe cases of psychosis. On that occasion he exhibited very loose associations, a key sign of schizophrenia. When I saw him the first time in January 1992, he had been in the SHU for about six months, and he was to remain there for several more months.

At our second interview at the medical facility in October 1992, this man seemed to be quite a bit less disturbed, and said he enjoyed being in an outpatient psychiatric setting. He did not seem agitated, his gaze was not bizarre, and he did not seem to be overmedicated. I reviewed his medical chart and discovered that he was taking much lower doses of antipsychotic medications compared to what had been prescribed while he was in the SHU. Interviewing this man a second time in a less harsh environment, it seemed quite evident to me that the SHU environment had been exacerbating his psychotic condition, and that while he was in the SHU his medication dosages were continually elevated in an attempt to keep up with the stress-induced symptoms. The higher medication dosages in the SHU caused side effects, including somnolence and slurred speech. A few months after my January visit he was transferred to the medical facility (having spent a year in solitary confinement) and was permitted out of his cell for supervised socialization. In this friendlier environment, his symptoms diminished markedly and he was able to get by on much less medication—and this was the reason for his much improved mental status when I interviewed him the second time.

---

I have mentioned three big reasons that so many prisoners suffer from serious psychiatric disorders: traumatic pasts, overcrowding and other harsh prison conditions, and confinement in psychosis-inducing supermaximum security units. In many of the worst cases of mental disorder I have seen, these three factors are additive. The typical prisoner suffering from a serious mental disorder in a supermaximum control unit reports massive trauma during his or her early years, an incapacity to tolerate life in a crowded prison without breaking rules and getting into fights, and a tendency for the extreme conditions of solitary confinement to trigger more extreme symptomatology and lead to even more desperate acting out and an even longer term in solitary confinement.

The prisoners who are least able to tolerate trauma are traumatized the most, and the result, in a shocking number of cases, is severe psychiatric breakdown and disability. The human damage is compounded when the mental health services are inadequate. In the next chapter I discuss the dreadful lack of quality mental health services in most prison systems.

3

# The Failure of Current Mental Health Programs

While the prison population has grown by leaps and bounds in recent decades, and the proportion of severely and chronically mentally disordered prisoners has enlarged rapidly, the budget for mental health services in correctional facilities has not expanded apace. As a result, there are many mentally disordered prisoners who take psychiatric medications but receive inadequate monitoring and none of the auxiliary treatments that are known to be essential if psychopharmacology is to be effective.

In preparation for expert testimony in *Coleman* v. *Wilson*, a class action lawsuit brought in 1993 by California prisoners claiming they were denied adequate mental health services, I interviewed a mentally disturbed male prisoner in the general population of Pelican Bay State Prison (PBSP). I described "Inmate #500" (the prisoners were assigned numbers in the interest of confidentiality) in a written declaration:

> Inmate #500, who seems to me a reliable historian, claimed that he would like to be in a mental health treatment program. He told me he had only been sent to PBSP because he received 115's (disciplinary write-ups) following his suicide attempts, otherwise he would have been eligible for a lower security level, and might have been sent to an institution where he could receive

> mental health treatment [almost no psychiatric treatment was available at PBSP at the time].
>
> During the two months Inmate #500 had been at PBSP he had put in two ducats to see the psychiatrist, but had not been seen at the time of his interview, nor had he received any psychotropic medications. As a result, he was hearing voices again and felt very paranoid. He explained that he stays in his cell most of the time because his mind drifts and this makes him very vulnerable: "Yesterday I missed a yell (from a guard with a rifle) to get down and almost got shot."
>
> His life was quite constricted. He ate only one meal per day in the dining room because he was frightened of being with other inmates, he stayed in his cell as much as he was able, and he was receiving no treatment of any kind. Social isolation and unabated symptomatology of the kind Inmate #500 exhibited are known to be very destructive for a mentally disordered person. Instead, he needs aggressive treatment and a safer environment, where he might feel free to stop isolating himself and begin to socialize with others and learn the skills of daily living he will need to cope with life in prison and life after prison.

Some mentally disordered prisoners try to cope in the general population and avoid victimization. Others are prone to suicide. Another large population of prisoners suffer from serious mental disorders but never come to the attention of the mental health staff. They merely vegetate in their cells or repeatedly get involved in altercations, the result being a term in punitive lock-up where their condition deteriorates further. A smaller number of prisoners, whose condition deteriorates to the point where they are flagrantly psychotic or suicidal, are transferred to a more intensive psychiatric treatment facility.

I have found prison medical and mental health treatment staffs generally conscientious and professional, but there is little they can do for the bulk of mentally disordered prisoners. So they focus on the small proportion of disturbed prisoners they can identify and offer some treatment, and they learn to live with the inadequacies of the program. Many treatment staff suffer burnout. They either leave correctional psychiatry or they become increasingly insensitive to the plight of the prisoners. Instead of standing up for their patients' therapeutic needs when the security staff order a strictly punitive response to a disturbed patients' rule-breaking, they stop protesting and begin following the directives of the security staff mechanically, or begin looking the other way when the security staff do something they consider countertherapeutic and inhumane to a prisoner.

Although there are standards for assessing the quality of mental health services behind bars, few if any institutions supply adequate services. In most prison systems, mental health care is sorely lacking. The tragic result is the warehousing of a large number of mentally ill prisoners who are confined to their cells and medicated.

## The Quality of Mental Health Care

Nationwide minimal standards have been established for correctional mental health services. Most prison systems, especially in the dozens of states that have been sued by prisoners asserting violations of their constitutional right to adequate health and mental health care, are attempting to comply with the minimal standards. But in all the prison systems I have investigated, the mental health services fall far short of providing a minimally acceptable quality of care to the large number of mentally disordered inmates in need of psychiatric attention. Too little attention is given to identifying mentally disturbed inmates. There is a deplorable lack of access to inpatient facilities, and there are huge gaps in terms of "intermediate levels of care."

## Minimal Standards of Care

In *Ruiz* v. *Estelle*, a 1980 class action lawsuit, Texas prisoners sued the state for violating their constitutional rights by confining them in excessively harsh conditions and depriving them of adequate mental health care. The federal district court formulated six components of a minimally adequate mental health treatment program:

1. A systematic screening procedure
2. Treatment that entails more than segregation and supervision
3. Treatment that involves a sufficient number of mental health professionals to adequately provide services to all prisoners suffering from serious mental disorders
4. Maintenance of adequate and confidential clinical records
5. A program for identifying and treating suicidal inmates
6. A ban on prescribing potentially dangerous medications without adequate monitoring

There have been similar lawsuits in other states. The National Commission on Correctional Health Care, the U.S. Department of Justice, and the American Public Health Association each publish updated minimal standards for the provision of mental health services in correctional facilities. The standards mandate elements of treatment such as adequate screening and assessment, crisis intervention, outpatient services, inpatient services, the proper use of seclusion and restraint, policies regarding involuntary medications, suicide prevention programs, training for nonclinical staff in the basics of suicide prevention and mental health care, peer review, record keeping, and so forth.

The quality of care ordered by the courts and mandated in the published standards are designed to approximate "the standard of care in the community." Of course, as public mental health budgets continue to be slashed, it could be argued that the standard of care in the community has deteriorated in recent years. Some even argue that the care prisoners receive inside correctional facilities is better than the care provided to low-income and homeless people in the community. But this is not true. In the community, even if quality mental health care is not available to everyone, each individual is free to seek higher quality treatment in another facility or even in another city. In contrast, the prisoner cannot seek services elsewhere when he or she is dissatisfied. Besides, we are not trained as professionals to practice one kind of care for patients who can afford quality treatment and a more lax kind for indigent patients. There is a standard of adequate care that cuts across class lines, regardless of cutbacks in public mental health facilities.

It is difficult to generalize about all correctional mental health programs. Each has its idiosyncratic strengths and weaknesses. In every correctional mental health delivery system I have investigated, there have been well-meaning, competent clinicians and administrators who are proud of certain aspects of their programs but admit they feel frustrated in their attempts to provide quality comprehensive care. And I have met others who care little about the quality of services and the plight of prisoners.

Where resources for mental health services are scarce, only the most severely disturbed patients receive more than token clinical attention. Some program administrators apply almost all of their limited budget to develop a model inpatient psychiatric unit—they know how to manage a hospital ward, even if the task of supplying comprehensive mental health services to an entire prison population is unachievable. The inpatient program becomes a showcase, evidence that the corrections department cares and is trying very hard to run a high-quality treatment program.

It is much easier to show a visitor an efficiently run inpatient unit than it is to explain how the mental health dollars are spread throughout the system to make prison life more tolerable for a large number of nonhospitalized mentally ill prisoners. The problem is, relatively few prisoners gain access to the inpatient unit, and even those lucky enough to be admitted stay for a short time and then receive inadequate follow-up services after they are discharged.

Other administrators put the bulk of their limited resources into a model drug rehabilitation program, or a suicide prevention program, or some other admirable but very partial intervention strategy. That way they can at least feel they are doing something proficiently, and they are meeting the standards of adequate care somewhere.

## Screening and Identifying Disturbed Prisoners

When I began touring county jails twenty-five years ago, I was shocked to discover a large number of prisoner deaths, a disproportionate number occurring within hours or days of incarceration. Reasons given for the deaths included suicide, head trauma sustained during arrest, drug overdose, drug withdrawal, heart attack, and diabetic crisis. I determined that in almost every case, these deaths could have been prevented had adequate screening occurred when the prisoners were first admitted to the jail.

We already knew, from earlier research reports as well as an editorial in the *Journal of the American Medical Association*, that the incidence of jail suicide was many times that of the general population and that half the suicides occurred within the first twenty-four hours of incarceration. It should have been obvious that a certain number of arrestees who had been hit over the head with an officer's billy club would develop subdural hematomas, and even though they might not become unconscious immediately, the blood clot in their brain would probably grow in size and eventually kill them or cause permanent brain damage. Since a significant proportion of arrestees were known drug users, the possibility of overdose or life-threatening withdrawal reactions should have been considered by jail administrators. And medical crises such as heart attacks, strokes, bleeding ulcers, and diabetic coma have long been known to occur when individuals prone to these conditions are subjected to severe stress, such as arrest and incarceration. But nobody was paying attention to the medical and psychiatric condition of arrestees! The courts began to require medical and psychiatric screening upon admission to jail.

The American Medical Association and many state governments began to publish standards for the provision of health and mental health services in local detention facilities, including the requirement that screening occur at the time of admission to jail. The screening should include questions designed to rule out the possibility that the arrestee is suffering from a critical medical condition or is prone to suicide. A nonphysician could administer the screening questionnaire—usually an officer who had emergency medical training or a nurse's assistant would do so—but the assumption was that any suspicious answers would cause the arrestee to be examined more thoroughly by a physician.

Today most local jails provide psychiatric screening when detainees are admitted, and provisions are made to treat offenders who are ill or at risk. Mental Health staff are assigned to treat prisoners who are found to be suicidal or suffer from mental disorders. Although most of the professional staff try very hard to carry out their responsibilities with admirable commitment and competence, the overcrowding continues to be a big problem in jails. There are breakdowns in the organization of services and programs, the staffing is rarely adequate (and with the trend toward privatization of mental health services in local detention facilities, staffs are likely to be downsized even further), and there are too many seriously disturbed jail inmates for a caring but overworked staff to serve adequately.

Screening procedures are effective only if carried out in a consistent and conscientious manner. In one county where I was asked to testify about an in-custody death, the protocol for screening involved a questionnaire that a nursing assistant filled out for each arriving offender. A disheveled, agitated, middle-aged white male arrestee was unable to respond appropriately to the questions, so the nursing assistant left the interview form blank except for writing that he seemed to be intoxicated and unable to cooperate on account of agitation and confusion. He was sent to a cell, where he was later found dead. The autopsy showed that he died of a subdural hematoma, caused by a blow to the head that either preceded his arrest or was delivered by the arresting officers. The tragic point here is that the screener had enough information to alert a physician about this man's critical condition.

A screening examination is a method for identifying arrestees who require emergency attention. A paraprofessional can be relied upon to conduct such an examination only if there is confidence that she or he will refer a case to a more highly trained professional if and when there is reason to suspect an emergency situation. The fact that this man failed the initial screening—that is, he was too incoherent to answer the questions—should have caused the nursing assistant to alert a physician. If a physician had examined this man while he was still conscious, the presence of the subdural hematoma probably would have been detected and emergency surgery might have saved this man's life. The more general point is that even procedures that are established to ensure quality care can break down under the stress of budget deficits and overcrowding, and often there are tragic consequences.

In prison, screening is less the issue. Rather, a thorough assessment of each incoming prisoner must be carried out to determine whether there is a medical or psychiatric condition that warrants attention. This assessment is usually accomplished at a reception center within the prison system, where new prisoners are sent until they can be classified in regard to security level and assigned to a specific institution and cellblock. Again, it is a very good idea to send new convicts to a reception center, but in almost every prison system I have toured, the system has run into major difficulties. In some prisons, crowding of the entire system causes a backlog in the reception center, requiring the housing of newly arrived convicts in impromptu dormitories set up in gymnasiums or dayrooms.

One problem with this arrangement is that prisoners of all security levels are housed together in a situation where the security staff is outnumbered and unable to intervene quickly when violence erupts. Many mentally disturbed prisoners in reception centers complain that they are repeatedly victimized by tougher inmates who will eventually be assigned to a higher security facility. But in the reception center, the staff have not figured out that the mentally ill convict needs protection and mental health services, or that the tougher predators need to be segregated. The more crowding there is, the less attention the staff can pay to altercations between prisoners, and the longer it takes to determine the needs of each prisoner.

Even after a prisoner has been assigned to a prison and a security level, he encounters difficulties in gaining access to mental health services. In part this is because it is unclear in a prison setting which symptoms qualify a prisoner for a psychiatric diagnosis. In a psychiatric hospital in the community, when an inmate saves excrement to make a bomb he can throw at a perceived enemy, the staff assumes he is acutely psychotic. But in prison, especially in a supermaximum control unit, the slinging of excrement is an everyday occurrence.

Similarly, if a mental patient in the community is terrified of leaving his or her room, there is the assumption that he or she suffers some degree of agoraphobia or paranoia. But in prison, many inmates stay in their cells all day because they are afraid their enemies will attack them out on the yard. And how is one to understand the diagnostic significance of sleeping all day in a dark cell—is it a sign of depression, or a very clever and intentional strategy for survival in a hostile prison world?

It is not easy to assess psychiatric disability in a prison setting, either. Most state laws outlining the criteria for involuntary hospitalization include the requirement that a mentally disordered person be a danger to self or others, or be unable to take care of himself or herself. If a police officer or mental health crisis team finds a man roaming the streets in rags and muttering incoherently to himself, and then escorts him home only to find a filthy apartment with an empty refrigerator, the criterion "not able to take care of himself" is met and the man is carted off to a psychiatric facility. But in prison, where an inmate is housed in a cell, fed in his cell, and ordered to take a shower every few days, what it means for him to be incapable of caring for himself is more difficult to determine. It is my impression that because prisoners are housed in cells and fed regularly, correctional psychiatrists tend to relax their guard when it comes to declaring a mentally disordered prisoner incapable of caring for himself.

Screening and early detection of mental disorders are crucial parts of any mental health treatment program, because the longer a severe mental disorder is left untreated, the more severe the symptomatology and the worse the prognosis. For instance, a large body of clinical research demonstrates that the quicker effective treatment is instituted for an acute schizophrenic episode, the shorter the duration of the episode and the better the prognosis. This is the rationale for the rapid administration of antipsychotic medications and the utilization of brief, intensive group and individual psychotherapy during a short stay in a psychiatric hospital. It is also recommended that the brief hospitalization be followed by longer term psychosocial rehabilitation, including case management, day treatment, and, if necessary, a nonhospital residential program in the community. When psychotic symptoms, including hallucinations, disordered thinking, and bizarre behaviors, are left untreated or undertreated for any length of time, the eventual prognosis is much worse than it would have been had adequate treatment been instituted in a timely fashion.

Psychiatrists of different persuasions explain this empirical finding very differently. Psychodynamically oriented practitioners and community psychiatrists claim that rapid treatment prevents the learning of bad habits, for instance the habits of acting bizarrely, viewing oneself as a mental patient, and becoming accustomed to others viewing one as a mental patient. Biological psychiatrists focus more on the likelihood that acute chemical abnormalities in the brain that produce the psychotic symptoms become fixed and more difficult to reverse over time. In any case, there is broad consensus among psychiatrists that when psychosis is left untreated for an extended period, or when the psychotic individual is repeatedly traumatized by stressful living conditions, the patient's condition is likely to deteriorate further and the psychosis is much more likely to become chronic.

In contrast to what happens to someone who suffers an acute psychiatric decompensation or breakdown in the community, when a prisoner begins to decompensate "inside," it takes longer than it would on the outside for his or her condition to be noticed and treated. The disturbed prisoner might be noticed by other prisoners and victimized before the staff can identify a mental disorder as the root of the problem, especially if the acute episode occurs in an overcrowded reception center. Often the prisoner has to scream for help or create a disturbance before treatment is instituted, but even then the screaming and ruckus-making are likely to be viewed by staff as manipulations, so the disturbed felon is very likely to be transferred to a lock-up setting as punishment instead of being sent to see a psychiatrist.

## Access to Intensive Services

Emergency psychiatric services and acute inpatient wards are a part of most prison systems, and they are a critical part of any mental health treatment program. Some state systems contract acute services out to a local psychiatric hospital or a nearby university facility. In many states the department of corrections has a contract with the department of mental health to run the inpatient units in the prisons. Some of these inpatient units are comparable to public psychiatric facilities outside prison walls.

The problem is access to care. Inpatient units or psychiatric wards within correctional systems tend to be small relative to the needs of the overcrowded prisons. For instance, while there might be 60,000 or 100,000 prisoners in a state correctional system, the single psychiatric inpatient facility might contain 75 or 150 beds. This means there is pressure on the staff to discharge patients quickly and make room for new admissions. It also means there is a backlog of patients elsewhere in the prison system waiting for a bed to become available in the inpatient unit.

By the time a prisoner who is experiencing an acute psychotic episode or a severe suicidal crisis is finally admitted to an inpatient facility, he or she may have spent weeks or months locked in a prison cell awaiting transfer. Then, after a week or two, the prisoner will probably be discharged from the inpatient unit and sent back to a nontreatment cellblock.

I have toured prisons where a dozen or more acutely psychotic inmates are confined to their cells twenty-four hours per day while they wait for approval to be transferred to the inpatient unit. The security staff do not know how to interact with them, so they ignore them except to bring them their food trays. The prisoners are usually seen for a few minutes each day by a harried psychiatrist and given strong antipsychotic medications, but they receive no other treatment. Nobody talks to them at any length, and they are left alone with their hallucinated voices, their terror, and their rage.

The disturbed prisoners who are fortunate enough to be transferred to the inpatient unit undergo more rigorous treatment, including group therapy and ward milieu meetings, and the professional staff spend time talking to them and adjusting their medications to better control their psychotic symptoms. But then, as soon as they seem stable, they are discharged from the only place where anyone paid them any sustained attention, and they find themselves in a prison cell once again.

Many severely disturbed prisoners report that they cycled through a prison psychiatric hospital once or twice, usually for a brief stay. The inpatient program becomes a showcase, evidence that the corrections department cares and is trying very hard to run a high-quality psychiatric treatment program.

## Intermediate Levels of Care

Where a large proportion of the limited funding for correctional mental health programs is put into a psychiatric inpatient unit, there is an unfortunate tendency to economize on "intermediate levels of care"—the services provided to prisoners whose mental disorders do not currently qualify them for admission to the inpatient unit but still make it difficult for them to cope in the mainline or general population.

In the community, the "intermediate level of care" is provided by an interacting web of outpatient clinics, day treatment programs, residential programs such as halfway houses, case managers, and vocational training programs. The idea is to help the mental patient learn the "skills of daily living" so he or she can live in the community, comply with his or her medication regimen, and avoid further hospitalizations. In prison, however, where the prisoners are forced to sleep in cells and remain within the institution, it makes little sense to talk of outpatient or residential programs. But even here the mentally disordered still need intermediate services. For instance, they need to meet in groups with trained mental health practitioners where they can learn how to manage their anger and all the daily assaults and dilemmas that are part of prison life. They need help understanding their mental conditions and realizing why they will do better if they comply with the medication regimen that has been designed for them. They may need some protection from perpetrators who victimize mentally disordered prisoners, but they may not want to go into "protective custody." In other words, they need a whole spectrum of services in order to stay out of trouble and avoid future breakdowns. But these are the services that are usually lacking in prison mental health treatment programs, and this is why a large number of mentally ill prisoners recycle into inpatient units and security housing units.

The psychiatrist in the Security Housing Unit at Wabash Valley Correctional Institution in Indiana informed me that approximately half of the prisoners in the SHU were suffering from a serious psychiatric disorder. They rarely talk to anyone except their neighbors, and even then they have to yell to be heard. Most of the mentally disordered inmates I interviewed in this facility were actively psychotic, or their psychotic symptoms were under tenuous control with antipsychotic or mood regulating medications.

I told the psychiatrist in charge that I believed these patients should not be housed in a control unit because that environment worsens their psychiatric condition. He did not disagree, but he explained that he is not in charge of assigning prisoners to cellblocks, and these men repeatedly get into trouble out in the general population. He described a pattern: They break enough rules to be sent to the SHU, he gives them enough medication while they are inside the SHU for them to settle down, but when they are released from the SHU back to the general population they are so angry about having been locked up in the SHU, and so unaccustomed to social interactions after spending time in isolation, that they begin to break rules again. Meanwhile, they vow to defy authority wherever they can, so they stop taking their medications. Eventually they are sent back to the SHU, psychotic and uncontrollable.

There is an inpatient psychiatric facility in another prison within the system, but it does not have enough beds to retain psychotic prisoners for an extended stay. And there are no intermediate level facilities where this psychiatrist can send mentally ill prisoners who are ready to leave the control unit but are incapable of coping in a mainline cellblock without some form of supportive psychotherapy. So the recycling continues unabated.

## The Uses of Medications

It is possible to control psychotic symptoms temporarily, for instance hallucinations, by merely medicating a person with strong antipsychotic agents. But this is far from adequate treatment. Rather, a person in an acute psychotic decompensation must be monitored closely and offered a variety of therapeutic modalities, including group and individual therapy, occupational or art therapy, a ward milieu, social work intervention aimed at improving some of the familial and social precipitants of the crisis, psychoeducation designed to teach the patient about the illness and the rationale of treatment, and so forth. Otherwise the medications merely control the symptomatic behavior by sedating the patient without dealing with the underlying anxieties and conflicts. The patient merely learns to mask the symptoms with high-dosage medications, and has not really learned anything about the illness or the importance of medications. Consequently, he is likely to stop complying with treatment as soon as he is given the choice to do so, and then the risk of relapse is quite high.

This is why a person suffering from a psychotic breakdown is hospitalized. People who are deemed to pose a high risk of suicide are hospitalized to protect them, and while they are hospitalized and being given intensive therapeutic attention, the reasons for their suicidal intentions are explored and, one hopes, sufficiently resolved that they'll not attempt suicide anew as soon as they leave the hospital. To merely medicate and isolate such a person is insufficient treatment. Antidepressant medications require weeks to take action, and the isolation actually increases the risk that, once out of the isolation cell, the person who is intent on self-destruction will proceed to take his life.

In correctional settings, where mental health clinicians have too many severely disturbed prisoners in their caseloads, the tendency is to sacrifice the activities that involve time, such as talking to patients in a confidential and trust-inducing setting. In most correctional institutions, the average prisoner/patient sees a psychiatrist for a few minutes once every month or two. The psychiatrist's assignment is to monitor the medications and order blood tests, for instance to determine a Lithium level or to check liver function if the medications have the potential of causing liver damage. In the supermaximum units I have toured, prisoners are not free to go to the clinic, so a psychiatrist makes "rounds" one or more times per week. Usually this means the psychiatrist walks along the ranges of cells and asks each prisoner how he is managing. Very few prisoners opt to do much talking.

There are also coercive abuses of medications behind bars. For instance, strong tranquilizers such as Thorazine and Haldol, designed for the treatment of psychotic conditions, are given by involuntary injection to disruptive but nonpsychotic prisoners to quiet them. Although these medications are effective at silencing the internal voices that command the schizophrenic prisoner to be assaultive, they are not very effective tranquilizers for nonpsychotic individuals. The dosage required to calm a nonpsychotic prisoner can put him to sleep or cause uncomfortable neurologic effects such as stiffness and muscle cramps.

Most states have laws and policies regarding the use of involuntary medications. Usually the procedure involves a hearing before a judge or review board to decide whether the prisoner is sane enough and has a right to refuse medications.

In many facilities I have toured the staff get around the requirement for a time-consuming hearing by coercing the prisoner into taking the medications. I have seen prisoners placed in four-and five-point restraints in their cells and told they will not be released, not even to use the toilet, until they agree to take the medications.

Guidelines for informed consent require that the physician inform the patient about the medication's effects and risks, and about alternative treatments. Violations of these guidelines occur with troubling frequency in all the prisons I have toured.

## Prisoners Deemed "Mad and Bad"

Most prison systems lack adequate treatment settings and programs for prisoners identified as "mad and bad." For instance, an inmate with a record of repeated violent episodes is likely to be refused admittance to a psychiatric program, even if he is acutely psychotic or suicidal, and even if in every one of his fights he was defending himself against prisoners who were harassing him on account of his mental illness. If he is fortunate enough to be admitted to an inpatient psychiatric ward, he is likely to be quickly discharged. Mental health staff explain that this group of prisoners are not motivated enough to benefit from treatment, and they are so disruptive they ruin the program for everyone.

Many of these prisoners get into fights in the general population or talk back to staff and land in security/isolation units. Alternatively, in an attempt to avoid seemingly inevitable confrontations and disciplinary write-ups, correctional staff order these prisoners to be "toplocked" (locked in their cells in a nonlock-up unit). Either in a lock-up unit or in a cell where they are toplocked, these prisoners are put on the psychiatrist's list for rounds. But since they are considered too disruptive to be in a group, they are unlikely to be included in any other kind of mental health treatment program. They vegetate in their cells, isolated and idle, where their rage grows and they become very regressed and incapable of participating in any kind of social interaction, even in the dayroom. Once prisoners are in lock-up, their subsequent inappropriate behaviors tend to be treated as disciplinary infractions rather than as signs of impending or acute mental decompensation.

There is merit in setting tough limits with disruptive prisoners, even ones suffering from severe mental disorders. It is impossible to supply psychiatric services in an unsafe situation. And mental health staff need to carefully avoid collusion in the dismissal of misconduct charges in cases where the prisoner is merely feigning a mental disturbance—and some of this kind of feigning does go on. At the same time, severely disturbed individuals are prone to act bizarrely and inappropriately because of their psychiatric condition.

Acting out and rule-breaking can be signs of a mental disorder that is not adequately treated and controlled. For instance, many disturbed prisoners hear voices or "command hallucinations" telling them to commit violence against themselves or others. When a psychotic prisoner loses control and follows the hallucinatory commands, more intensive treatment is needed. He might need a higher dose of antipsychotic medication, and he might need to be placed in a seclusion room until someone can talk to him to determine whether a precipitating event set him off. For instance, was he threatened or raped, or did he just receive news of a child who is in trouble on the outside?

Instead, there is a tendency in prison for the mental health staff to defer to security staff, who move in and lock up the disruptive prisoner. Mental health care is relegated to an afterthought. No one takes the time to talk to the prisoner or contact the family to determine whether there was a precipitating assault or a piece of bad news. And it is very difficult for mental health staff to gain the trust of a prisoner who has been locked in a cell and is screaming about the unfairness of it all. The result is a very angry prisoner in a cell, ready to unload his rage on anyone who is unlucky enough to come by. Of course, at that point, mental health staff tend to stay clear, claiming the prisoner is too angry and too recalcitrant to treat. The disturbed, disruptive prisoner is left alone with his psychotic delusions.

Of course, there are some individuals who will never be rehabilitated. They are the psychopaths and serial killers who create fear in the community and deserve to be quarantined for life. But they are a very small proportion of prisoners today. There is a much larger number of very disturbed individuals who become violent and uncontrollable only after being repeatedly traumatized in prison, and many of these people will be released some day. If the staff were to talk to these difficult-to-manage prisoners and slowly gain their trust, there would be opportunities down the road to redirect their energies into constructive projects that would help prepare them to resume their status as free citizens. I return to this subject in Chapter Ten.

Warehousing is something that happens by default. When treatment and rehabilitation programs are lacking, prisoners are left to their own devices. Mentally disturbed prisoners have a very difficult time remaining stable in the absence of safe, supervised social interactions and meaningful structured activities. Too many end up confined to their cells, where their condition deteriorates.

## Staff Attitudes

Aside from mandated tasks such as providing reports to courts and parole boards and providing court-ordered treatment for sex offenders, many correctional mental health staff have insufficient time to meet the demand for direct clinical services. After attending to the most serious cases of psychosis and the most imminent suicide risks, the harried staff have little patience with a prisoner they suspect may be manipulating them to get drugs or attention.

But the conscientious clinician has to believe she is accomplishing something at work. If she feels she is unable to give patients the care their conditions warrant because she has to see too many patients each day, or if security considerations prevent her from acting on her clinical judgment in too many cases, she tries to find a more limited aspect of clinical practice where she can exercise some degree of autonomy and control. An example of this kind of retreat into a delimited area of mastery is a psychiatrist I met who prides himself on keeping excellent clinical records.

In most of the prisons I have toured, clinical record-keeping has been quite deficient. Notes are sporadic. Inconsistency is pervasive, as each clinician sees a patient and alters the treatment without clearly spelling out the objective findings and the rationale for switching medications or housing assignments. The psychiatrist I met is an exception. The progress notes and orders he enters into charts are quite commendable. He notes the prisoner/patient's condition at the time of his visit, any alterations in the treatment plan he feels are indicated, and a date for the next clinic appointment.

The problem is that this psychiatrist does not have enough time to see all the prisoners who need attention, and his treatment strategy is limited to prescribing medications and confining disturbed prisoners to their cells. There are no other clinicians on staff in this prison, there is no group therapy, no social worker to contact the family, and no psychiatric rehabilitation program of any kind. In addition, security staff move patients to different tiers and cellblocks whenever they feel a transfer is indicated for security reasons, and they never consult the treating psychiatrist about the move or the reason for it. He confides:

> I'm not used to this kind of antitherapeutic program. Usually, when I have a patient in the hospital, I call the shots. I order a single room or a double room, and I order the patient be sent to a seclusion room when I decide the clinical situation calls for it. In this prison, I don't have control over any of that, and I can't even order supplemental services like a social worker contact with the family. And since I'm the only doc here and the prison's overfilled with a lot of disturbed cons, I only have a few minutes to see each patient. The only thing I have any control over is the quality of charting, so I make damn sure my notes are clear and concise.

## Staff Burnout

I have met correctional mental health staff who are very insensitive and uncaring, and cooperate with security staff in acts of outright cruelty toward prisoners. A much larger number seem very conscientious, competent, and caring and work very hard to provide adequate mental health services. They try to do good where they can, and at least to do no harm. But because the number of prisoners needing mental health services is huge, and most prisons' mental health delivery systems are underfunded, understaffed, and sadly lacking, the caring staff eventually begin to suffer from burnout.

The signs of burnout are omnipresent in correctional mental health programs today. I feel it when I talk to staff members. They are less than enthusiastic about their work. They complain about prison administrators and tell of bickering and rivalry at meetings.

There is high absenteeism and many vague complaints of illness, and there is low attendance at staff training events unless attendance is mandatory. Many staff members seem intent on isolating themselves and are uninterested in trying new approaches.

Privately, staff members say they feel stuck and unappreciated, and resent having to follow the orders and plans of security staff when their job is to provide mental health services. A clinical psychologist in a maximum security state prison told me: "I wasn't trained to be a cop. Just when I begin to gain a patient's trust, he gets in trouble with the guards and they move him to a segregation unit where I can't go see him anymore. And by the time the guy gets to segregation, he's so angry he won't talk to me anyway, and then all the gains we made in therapy are totally erased and he starts acting out all over the place." Many mental health staff wonder why they remain in a correctional setting and search for ways to leave.

Maslach and Leiter point out that burnout occurs among those who do "people work" of some kind. They identify three dimensions of burnout: exhaustion, cynicism, and ineffectiveness. They explain that burnout is not a problem of workers lacking the strength or will to carry on with the work, rather it is a problem of the social environment. If the workplace does not recognize "the human side of work," then the risk of burnout is high.

The Maslach Burnout Inventory is a structured interview wherein staff are asked anonymously whether a series of statements fit their experience. For instance: "I feel used up at the end of the workday." "I've become more callous toward people since I took this job." "I deal very effectively with the problems of my recipients." The inventory can be used to help the staff begin to talk among themselves about what is ailing them at work. When I ask correctional mental health staff these questions, the replies suggest widespread burnout.

The more burned out the staff become, the more they distance themselves from any involvement on a feeling level with the prisoners' plight. After all, caring about the prisoners makes the job that much more difficult, especially when the caring professional is unable to halt what he or she considers inappropriately brutal interventions on the part of security staff, or when the administration makes it very clear it does not approve of professional staff making waves.

A certain degree of independence from security staff is required if mental health staff are to provide humane treatment. Of course, security is a primary consideration in penal institutions. Mental health staff must work closely with security staff to maintain safety inside the institution and collaborate on a management plan for disturbed prisoners. But too often security staff call all the shots, even when a prisoner's actions are clearly the result of his or her psychiatric condition and the prisoner poses no imminent safety risk.

## Fears About Being Manipulated

Prisoners can be very manipulative, and many do feign mental illness. In a certain number of cases, it is a survival tactic. A reputation as a "crazy" can be a protective device: Other prisoners stay clear of a known "crazy" because they cannot predict how he will react. Some prisoners feign mental illness in order to gain a transfer to a more tolerable housing assignment. If one is afraid of tougher prisoners, or unable to tolerate the loneliness of prison life, the programs designed for mentally disabled prisoners appear relatively inviting. Other prisoners feign mental illness because they think being identified as mentally ill will help them win a lighter sentence, gain a new trial, or in some other way improve their legal situation. Still others merely seek attention. So correctional mental health professionals do need to distinguish between prisoners who are feigning mental illness and prisoners who actually suffer from a serious disorder.

But that is not always easy to do. Many prisoners suffer from a serious mental illness *and* feel a need to manipulate in order to get the attention they need. And often they are absolutely right about the need to manipulate. There is a vicious cycle: The more insufficient the mental health services and the more intent the staff are on denying services to prisoners who might be manipulating, the more the truly mentally impaired felon is forced to manipulate if she is to get the care she needs. For instance, the disturbed felon might have to make a commotion or hit someone in order to gain the attention of the mental health staff.

Mental health workers who are too intent on identifying the manipulators tend to miss this nuance and deny these prisoners the care they need. In the prisons I have investigated, a prisoner is perceived either as a manipulator, in which case all her needs tend to be neglected, or as a bona fide mental patient. Of course, discrimination on the part of staff is required. The few slots available for intensive treatment should not be filled by the prisoners who are the most sophisticated manipulators. But the capacity to discriminate in this regard is part of a mental health clinician's art, inside or outside the walls.

## Insufficient Postrelease Planning

Over 90 percent of prisoners, including those with severe and persistent mental disorders, will eventually serve their full sentence and be released. In many states, they are set loose with little or no planning for treatment or support services on the outside. This makes postrelease adjustment difficult for the most stable ex-felon, but for those suffering from severe mental disorders, especially if they have served a significant proportion of their prison term in lock-up of some kind, successful adjustment is improbable. The recidivism rate for all ex-prisoners three years after release is 63 percent; for ex-prisoners suffering from serious mental disorders it is over 80 percent.

Some correctional mental health staff try to talk to case managers in the county to which the mentally disordered prisoner is being released in order to set up a postrelease treatment plan. But in recent years the treatment, training, and vocational opportunities available to ex-felons have shrunk dramatically, just as treatment and rehabilitation opportunities inside have diminished. And mentally disordered prisoners who have been warehoused in their cells for most of their fixed terms, especially if they have no family to return home to, tend to get into serious trouble immediately after they are released.

For instance, I interviewed a very psychotic prisoner in an administrative segregation unit who had been released several months earlier at the expiration of a fixed prison term, only to wait in the parking lot for a nurse he "had a crush on" to leave work and rape her. He was caught immediately, and found to be hearing voices that commanded him to commit the rape. After conviction for the rape he was returned to prison to serve a much longer sentence.

In some cases, a mentally disordered prisoner who has served his time is transferred directly from prison to a noncorrectional treatment facility. Too often the procedure is very poorly planned. For instance, the director of mental health for a county that contains a high-security prison told me the story of a disturbed, violent patient whom the state prison foisted on her department without any advance notice. She received a call late one Friday afternoon from the assistant warden at the prison, informing her they were about to release a male prisoner who was clearly psychotic and out of control. She asked why he was being released at the prison gate instead of being sent back to the county where he had been convicted, and was informed that he had no family and had committed crimes in several counties.

The assistant warden added: "So I guess he's yours to deal with as you see fit." Then he gave her this unsolicited advice: "If I were you, I'd call the sheriff and have him arrange to send some officers over to the prison gate in an hour, when we release this guy, and pick him up on the assumption he is mentally ill and a danger to others." She did what he advised, the sheriff's deputies intercepted the released prisoner and transported him to the county's psychiatric emergency room. Even though he was taking high doses of antipsychotic medications, the emergency room psychiatrist felt he was hallucinating, delusional, and a clear danger to others because of his propensity to act out violently at the slightest provocation. He had to be admitted to a locked psychiatric unit.

Many other prisoners suffering from serious mental disorders are simply released at the end of their fixed sentences and given a one-way bus ticket to a destination of their choice within the state. Depressed prisoners tend to leave prison quietly, but many of them suffer from an emotional paralysis caused by too much time alone in a cell, and have great difficulty returning to their families, looking for work, and beginning life anew on the outside.

A growing number of mentally ill and chronically disruptive ("mad and bad") prisoners serve the final years of their fixed sentences in a supermaximum security unit. Then, because the law mandates they be set free, they "max out of the SHU" right onto the streets. They are ill-prepared for life in the community. Many are re-arrested very quickly, but only after they commit new crimes. Obviously this kind of recycling imperils public safety.

---

A term in prison is traumatic under any circumstances for convicts who are susceptible to emotional breakdowns. But certain features of prison life today are especially stressful and cause damage far beyond what would be expected in a well-run prison setting. These include pervasive racism, inattention to the special needs of women, sexual harassment by staff, the horror of rape, staff insensitivity toward rape victims, lack of quality contact with loved ones, and a frighteningly high incidence of suicide behind bars. In Part II I focus on these extremely traumatic, and in many instances preventable, circumstances and events.

# PART II

# What Goes on Behind Bars

# 4

# Racism: A Mental Health Hazard

Racial discrimination in arrests and sentencing leads to stark racial disparity in the composition of the prison population. Guards, most of them white, have a degree of authority over their wards that is unparalleled in society outside the walls. All social interactions tend to be viewed through the prism of race. In an environment where racial lines are so obvious, and where harsh conditions are the rule, the issue of race becomes the nidus around which tensions constellate and trouble erupts.

Blatant and unopposed racism has devastating effects on the mental health of prisoners. Quite a few prisoners of color are driven mad by the racism and their lack of recourse. To add injury to insult, there is racial discrimination in the very interpretation of madness, and black prisoners who become angry and suffer emotional breakdowns are more likely than their white counterparts to be thrown in the hole and denied adequate mental health treatment.

## Race Relations in Prison

Racial lines are drawn sharply in prison. A large majority of prisoners are people of color. Since most prisons are built far from urban centers and employ many local residents, a large percentage of prison staff are whites who have relatively little experience relating to people of color. Where brutality occurs, it is very likely to be viewed as racially motivated. Although determining precisely which charges are well-founded is often difficult, there is sufficient evidence to confirm the overall impression that racism is a huge problem. But hearing officers and appeal panels are mainly composed of white staff, and prisoners complain it's all very unfair.

## Racial Disparity in Sentencing

Racism permeates the criminal justice system. People of color are more likely than whites to be stopped by police, to be searched, to be arrested, to be defended by a public defender with a huge caseload, to be convicted, and to be given a harsh sentence. Over 30 percent of African-American males between the ages of twenty and twenty-nine were under criminal justice supervision in 1994—inside jails and prisons or on probation or parole.

In some urban areas, the figures are even more startling. For instance, 42 percent of black men between the ages of eighteen and thirty-five in Washington, D.C. are under criminal justice supervision on any given day, and the comparable figure in Baltimore is 56 percent. African Americans are incarcerated at a rate of 1,947 per 100,000 African-American citizens, compared to a rate of 306 per 100,000 for white citizens. Blacks already constitute over 50 percent of the prison population, Hispanics another 15 percent. Native Americans are vastly overrepresented in the prison population. The National Criminal Justice Commission calculates that in the year 2020, 33.3 percent of African Americans and 25.6 percent of Hispanics between the ages of eighteen and thirty-four will be incarcerated.

The disproportion grows as the level of punishment becomes more severe. The Center on Juvenile and Criminal Justice in San Francisco reports that in the first two years that California's three-strikes law was in effect, 43 percent of those sentenced for a third strike were African American, even though they make up only 7 percent of the state population and 20 percent of those arrested. And 40 percent of occupants of death rows nationwide are black.

In Pennsylvania, 131 out of 210 prisoners on death row are black, or 62 percent.

The racial disproportion in sentencing has accelerated rapidly since the mid-1980s and the declaration of a "war on drugs." Whereas the incarceration rate in state prisons on drug charges rose 306 percent for whites between 1985 and 1995, it rose 707 percent for African Americans.

It is not difficult to understand why this is the case. For instance, federal legislation designates sentences five times as harsh for possession or sale of crack cocaine compared to sentences involving powder cocaine. Ninety percent of those arrested nationwide for possession of crack cocaine are African Americans, whereas 75 percent of those arrested for powder are white. And eight out of ten crack cocaine cases in federal court involve African Americans, whereas the comparable figure in powder cocaine cases is 33 percent. Although African Americans are less than 13 percent of the total population, and approximately 13 percent of those arrested for drug possession, they are 55 percent of those convicted of drug possession and 74 percent of the total serving sentences for possession.

## Racial Tensions "Inside"

The proportion of people of color in the prison population has been rising for many decades. In 1930, 75 percent of all prison admissions were white and 22 percent were African American; in 1992, 29 percent of prison admissions were white, whereas 51 percent were African American and 20 percent were Hispanic.

Within the prisons, the proportion of people of color rises with the security level. Minimum security prisons contain disproportionately more whites whereas maximum security prisons contain more people of color. Inhabitants of protective custody units tend to be disproportionately white whereas the supermaximum security units contain up to 90 or 95 percent blacks and Latinos.

Race is the defining characteristic of individuals and groups behind bars. Voluntary segregation by race is usually unspoken but mandatory. Young felons tell me that even though they had close friends of different races on the streets, when they entered prison they quickly learned to stay with their own race. As one young prisoner explains: "It's dangerous to associate with other races, even with people you knew back on the streets."

One is struck immediately by the strict racial segregation on the yards of maximum security prisons. Black prisoners are lifting weights in one corner of the yard, whites in another, and the Latinos are gathered in still another area, talking or kicking a soccer ball. Whenever tensions mount and a fight seems imminent, the stragglers and loners who were wandering around the yard alone or in pairs quickly join the largest group of their own race they can reach. Many mentally disordered prisoners get into trouble because they are unable to sense the imminence of racial strife and to join the right group.

In a supermaximum control unit in Indiana, I spoke to a white prisoner who sported a KKK tattoo on his forearm. He told me: "I don't really have anything against blacks. I just think it's better if we all stick to our own people. But I think this racism thing works both ways. There's a black cop on the morning shift who's in charge of letting us out on the yard, and he always makes the white guys go to the yard early in the morning so if we want to sleep in we have to give up our yard time. But he sends the black guys to the yard later in the day so they can sleep in *and* get their yard time. It's little things like that that keep whites and blacks mad at each other." In fact, there are only two or three African-American officers in this particular unit, and several dozen white officers. But the point is that race matters very much, to everyone.

The racial dynamics can be subtle. For instance, one white prisoner told me of incidents in which a certain officer was more lenient with a white or a black, the other inmate assumed it was because of race, the two began to fight, and the officer wrote both of them tickets for infractions of the rule against fighting. In one prison I visited in Michigan, there are two serving lines in the general population cafeteria. The unspoken rule is that blacks go through one and are served by blacks, and whites go through the other to be served by whites. Inevitably, the blacks complain the servings are larger in the white line, and the whites complain the servings are larger in the black line.

Racial discrimination can also be quite obvious, mirroring society-wide race relations. For instance, in many prisons the jobs and industry assignments that are highest paying—for example, carpentry, tool and die, machine maintenance—are filled to a very great extent by white inmates, whereas those that are less prestigious, less well-paying, and less valuable in terms of training for postrelease jobs—for example, cafeteria, porter, and janitorial positions—are filled disproportionately by minority inmates. White inmates learn skills and tend to be in supervisory positions, while blacks and other minorities tend to be assigned more menial work and to be lower in the status hierarchy—if they are working at all (remember, a greater proportion are in security segregation).

Racist attitudes on the part of guards can cause intense emotional conflict and strife in prisoners of color. For example:

> A black prisoner in a minimum security facility routinely passes through the front gate of the prison to do his job grooming the prison grounds. He leaves, works, and reenters under the direct supervision of a black guard who is responsible for his work crew. When he reenters the gate, he is put through a metal detector, pat-searched, and permitted to pass. One day there is a new, white guard on duty when he reenters the prison following a work shift, and the newcomer orders him to strip, bend over, and spread his buttocks.
>
> He tells the officer that he passes through the gate every day, and is never out of sight of a staff member while he is outside, so there is no need to go through that procedure. The prisoner's supervisor stepped down the hall for a moment, so the prisoner is alone with the new guard. The guard stiffens and says through clenched teeth: "Boy, are you refusing to follow an order?"

> The prisoner later tells me: "It's all I could do to keep myself from decking the guy. That racist cop was just trying to put me down, humiliate me so I'd know who was the master. I came this close (he gestures with two fingers representing a very small space) to clocking him—that would have landed me in the hole for a really long spell. Finally I submitted to the exam."

The man who told me this story was emotionally stable. But what if he had been someone with an intermittent emotional disorder who knew that the only way he could avoid falling into a downward spiral of rage, ego disintegration, and subsequent delusions was to avoid all interactions that might provoke his anger. There would have been no way for him to avoid this ugly interaction with the guard, and very likely his mental stability would have been jeopardized.

White officers have many unofficial ways of discriminating against prisoners of color. For instance, when the team from Human Rights Watch, of which I was a part, toured the Security Housing Unit at the Wabash Valley Correctional Institution in Indiana in July 1997, we discovered a black prisoner confined in a cell covered with racist graffiti. Racist epithets such as "White Power" were printed on the walls in large letters, and the words "Fuck all Niggers" was etched into the mirror. There was a drawing of a hooded Klansman over the bed, along with a large swastika. Obviously, this kind of treatment negatively affects a prisoner's mental health, especially if he is at all prone to paranoia. The cell's occupant told us he had been transferred to this cell six days earlier, following an argument he had with a white guard. The team asked prison officials about the situation and were told that the prisoner was transferred to that cell because it was the only one available at the time.

Of course not every guard is a racist, and prisoners of color are quick to admit that some guards are very fair. They complain, however, that the code among correctional officers makes it very difficult for the "good cops" to interfere when a "bad cop" is harassing or brutalizing a prisoner. I am told of incidents in which a white officer arbitrarily picks a fight with a black prisoner, the prisoner makes some attempt to defend himself or ward off the blow, the white officer proceeds to pummel the black prisoner, and a black officer who is witnessing the entire episode is unable to do anything to halt the racist attack.

In the prisons I have toured, there has been little or no staff training about cultural diversity or interracial relationships, and the officers tend to be very unsophisticated in terms of race relations. Prisoners of color consistently complain that the white officers do not understand them and do not know how to talk to blacks and Latinos. They also feel that most of the staff look down on them and call them derogatory names. Where racism and interracial tensions are left to fester, inmates of all races are more at risk for attack, harassment, uncontrolled violent outbursts, and mental disturbances of all varieties.

## Race and Gangs

Prison gang-containment policies tend to increase racial tensions. Prison gangs don't keep membership lists. Security staff guess which prisoners are in gangs. They get tips from law enforcement agencies in the community, they observe associations between prisoners in the dayrooms and on the yards, and they have the word of informants. Then they make their guesses.

Of course, with a mostly white staff and a predominantly minority prison population, racial stereotypes come into play. Many white staff do not really understand the meaning of ritual handshakes or fully understand why certain people of color associate with each other. A black prisoner who is not gang-affiliated might associate with other blacks, including some known gang members, because it is safer to be with them than to cross the yard and enter territory controlled by Latinos or whites. And a black prisoner may banter with gang members and shake their hands only because they all grew up in the same neighborhood. But a white guard who does not know much about the prisoners' background is likely to conclude that the fraternizing and handshaking signify gang membership.

When a prisoner whom the guards accuse incorrectly of gang membership tells them he isn't gang-affiliated, the guards respond: "That's OK. If you're not in a gang, then you have to give us the name of someone who is, so we won't need to throw you into the SHU with them." If a prisoner informs on a gang member, there is grave danger of retaliation. Often a prisoner who opts to "snitch" will falsely identify a loner or a mentally ill prisoner who lacks the connections and capability necessary to retaliate.

I do not mean to imply that, were there a foolproof system for accurately identifying gang members, isolating them in supermaximum security units would be an effective strategy for controlling prison violence. I agree with the many criminologists who argue that this whole approach to gang-containment is badly flawed and counterproductive. One unfortunate consequence of policies aimed at quarantining gang members in supermaximum security units is that a large number of mentally disturbed prisoners inevitably wind up there, while many actual gang members are missed. But I will not explore the policy question here. My point for now is, when it comes to gang affiliation, racial stereotypes lead to many mistaken identifications.

Prisoners in supermaximum security units claim that white guards label prisoners of color as gang members without sufficient evidence. African-American and Latino prisoners tell me that white guards are afraid of tough men of color, and just as the police in their communities, they brutalize those they fear the most. Whether or not the charges of racist discrimination are justified in every individual case—a certain number of prisoners actually are gang members—it is quite clear that policies aimed at containing gangs serve to increase the proportion of people of color in the high-security and supermaximum units.

I have heard many accusations about guards inciting prisoners of one race or one gang to beat or kill prisoners of another race or gang. It is always the prisoners' word against the guards'. But sometimes evidence of abuse breaks into the news. For instance, *Sixty Minutes* ran a video on March 30, 1997, showing the guards at maximum security Corcoran State Prison in California forcing two black and two Latino prisoners into a prison yard where, since they were known members of rival gangs, they would have to fight. It is alleged that some of the guards at Corcoran, with the implied consent of superiors, purposely released sworn enemies into the yard at the same time, even though they knew the prisoners would have to fight to the death, and bet on the outcome.

One inmate gladiator who won eleven staged fights told Dr. Corey Weinstein in an interview: "I was made aware by the officers that there was money riding on me to win, I was even thanked by officers for making them a bit richer." As soon as it became clear who had prevailed, the guards would order the inmates to cease and desist immediately. If the prisoners did not cease fighting immediately, the guards would shoot them. More than fifty inmates have been shot in this manner since the prison opened in 1988, and seven have died.

Two officers who were uncomfortable with the way prisoners were being forced to fight and die for the entertainment of the guards told their stories to the FBI. The California Correctional Police Officers Association and the California Department of Corrections responded to the charges, claiming the guards at Corcoran were merely following departmental policy and therefore were not guilty of misconduct. This is an important point. Often a corrections department fires a few malevolent officers after an incident that has the potential of damaging the department's reputation. By claiming the guards at Corcoran were merely following policy, in this instance a departmental directive issued in 1989 to desegregate the once segregated maximum security yards, correctional authorities open themselves to the very logical charge that it is their deliberate policies, and not merely the malevolence of individual guards, that leads to interracial strife and deaths on the yard. In February

1998, the U.S. Department of Justice indicted eight guards for violating the civil rights of prisoners at Corcoran.

## Lack of Recourse

Many stories I hear from prisoners go approximately like this: A black prisoner is beaten by one or several white officers. The officers charge the prisoner with refusing to follow an order and assaulting an officer. The prisoner complains he has been "jumped" by racist officers because he is black. The ruling by a panel of hearing officers goes against the prisoner. He is given a sentence in punitive segregation.

A panel of hearing officers drawn exclusively from prison staff tends to be a majority of white. This does not prove that the proceedings are racially biased. But as one prisoner recently told me: "How do we know these white cops and counselors don't just decide in advance that every black prisoner who comes before them is wrong just because the cop who wrote him up is white, and there'd be no way for me to protest that kind of racism or appeal their decision. They don't even let me bring in another prisoner as my witness or a lawyer to plead my case."

There certainly are times when a black prisoner attacks a white officer. But there are also cases where the officers beat a prisoner and then charge him with assaulting an officer in order to cover up the beating. If there was a fair disciplinary hearing process, we might expect the decision to go against the prisoner some of the time and against the correctional officer on other occasions. The fact is that in most prisons between 90 and 100 percent of the rulings go against the prisoners. One begins to wonder about the fairness of the procedure. More important, where there is a perception on the part of most prisoners that the hearing process is unfair and they have no real right to appeal, resentments about the racism inherent in the process tend to fester, and the mental health of prisoners suffers.

## The Emotional Costs of Racism

When black, Native American, and Latino prisoners enter prison and see mainly white staff in charge of so many people of color, they are reminded of their experiences in the community, including beatings they received at the hands of white police and the times they were hauled off to jail unfairly and charged with resisting arrest. Racial discrimination traumatizes the most stable prisoners, but in those prone to mental illness and suicide, the repercussions of racism include intensified mental deterioration and self-destructiveness.

### Fear, Rage, and Despair in Stable Prisoners

Black prisoners tell me they fear for their lives in a setting where mainly white guards have absolute control over their every move and there is no reprisal when a prisoner is killed or maimed by a brutal guard. This is certainly not to say all guards are racists, but incidents involving discrimination against prisoners of color are numerous enough to give these prisoners cause to fear racist abuse, and that fear creates psychiatric symptoms.

For instance, a black prisoner in his early thirties who has spent twelve years in prison and expects to be considered for parole in two more years tells me: "These fools [the guards] are totally in charge of my life—and they admit they hate blacks—the only way to survive is to say 'yessir' and let them run their games." I ask if the situation makes him nervous and he tells me:

> I get attacks. My heart starts pounding like it's going to break out of my chest, I can't breathe, I start to see lights, I get to where I feel like I'm gonna faint. I can't tell when it's going to happen. I never had attacks like this before coming here. I'm just always scared the cops [guards] are going to jack me up for something. There's no telling when they're gonna beat you, or even kill you.

> They beat up a cellie of mine so bad he's been in a wheelchair ever since. I'm just trying to do my time peacefully so I can get home in one piece.

Black prisoners tell me the daily humiliations of life in prison serve as constant reminders of slavery. They are treated like animals. They are bound in chains while being transported. Guards with shotguns stand over them. And if they protest when a racist guard calls them "nigger" or "boy," they risk a beating and a long sentence in solitary confinement.

Indeed, the Thirteenth Amendment freed the slaves, but it contained a clause permitting involuntary labor as punishment for a crime. Prior to the Civil War, Southern prisons contained very few African Americans because slave owners had the authority to discipline their slaves as they saw fit. But immediately following the abolition of slavery, a large number of ex-slaves were sent to prison, often for minor offenses. Plantation owners were permitted to lease black convicts to work their fields. In many cases, the arrangement was worse than slavery. Antebellum slave owners had an interest in maintaining the health of their slaves, but a plantation owner could work his leased convicts to death and then request replacements for those who became sick or died. And a huge number of black convicts died during Reconstruction from overwork, beatings, or exposure to the elements.

Prisoners of color report they feel extremely vulnerable, "very much like a slave." They know they have no recourse when they are victimized by racism. Some report feeling frustrated and rageful. Others say they experience intense despair. The common denominator is a sense that there is nothing they can do to alter their plight. Some become resigned to their fate. Either they maintain their sanity by staying in touch with family and community and planning for their eventual release, or lethargy sets in and they fall into depression. Others act out in impotent acts of defiance. Relatively stable prisoners report severe symptoms in response to racial discrimination, including anxiety, depression, panic attacks, phobias, nightmares, flashbacks, uncontrollable rage reactions, and so forth.

We know from research on PTSD that the negative effects of severe trauma are worsened by the victim's belief he was treated unfairly while being traumatized. A black prisoner had been sentenced by a prison disciplinary panel to a term in punitive detention as a result of an argument he had with a guard. He served the sentence in solitary confinement, and then he appealed the panel's ruling by suing the department of corrections in an outside court. I asked him why he was appealing the ruling to a court when he had already completed the term in solitary—did he want a financial settlement? He shook his head, no, and replied: "I just want them to admit it wasn't fair what that cop did to me—if they'd just admit that I wouldn't even mind having done all that time in the hole for nothin'."

## Emotional Breakdowns in Less Stable Prisoners

Prisoners who suffer from serious mental disorders have trouble coping in the best of environments. In prison they do not do well at all. And if they are black, Latino, or Native American, and there is a significant amount of racism in the institution, they are especially prone to decompensation.

There are many kinds of breakdowns. I highlight two that come to light often in my interviews with mentally disturbed prisoners of color:

1. Despair and hopelessness leading to depression
2. Mounting rage that brings on psychosis

The theme of hopeless resignation is widespread among prisoners of color who suffer from severe depression. "These rednecks are in charge, they don't like me because I'm black, and there's nothing I can do about it. They're never going to let me out of here." Again, it is a huge mistake to assume that all correctional staff are racist. There are many who pride themselves on their fairness and care about the well-being of the prisoners. But there are also "bad apples" in every barrel, and the occasional racist officer makes the daily lives of black and Latino prisoners quite miserable. Prisoners who are prone to depression, and see acts of racist oppression all around them but feel they have absolutely no recourse and no way to improve their predicament, are very likely to fall into depression.

Another kind of breakdown involves a growing rage leading to ego disintegration. Although most stable people get angry and get over it, some people who suffer from schizophrenia and other forms of psychosis have very fragile egos, and as they begin to get angry their ego starts to fall apart. The anger continues to mount as though feeding on itself, the prisoner regresses to ever more primitive behaviors, and his rage mounts as he loses contact with reality. When a black prisoner who is prone to this kind of self-destructive anger and ego disintegration is subjected to racist treatment while in prison, there is a good chance he'll decompensate and become psychotic.

It is very difficult to predict precisely which individuals will decompensate under a certain degree of stress, but among the mainly minority prisoners housed in supermaximum security units, there are a frighteningly large proportion of very angry and very psychotic individuals. When I talk with a prisoner from this group, I consistently hear the same story of progression into madness: The prisoner perceives that he is being abused. He feels the abuse is part of the racism that permeates the criminal justice system. He is quite convinced there is nothing he can do about it. He believes there is no longer anything to be gained by his following the rules and controlling his anger since nobody listens to him. The rage mounts. He loses control and gets into trouble. He is sent to solitary confinement where the idleness and isolation make him more rageful. And his mental condition deteriorates even further.

The details vary in each case, but even when a prisoner is quite delusional, it is possible to discern a kernel of truth about race relations at the center of his concerns. For example:

Mr. P., a tall, muscular, thirty-four-year-old African-American man, spent over half of his twelve years in prison confined in lock-up units. He spent time in a psychiatric hospital prior to being incarcerated, where he was assigned a diagnosis of paranoid schizophrenia. When I talked to Mr. P., he stood very erect and glared menacingly through the food slot in the solid door of his cell. When I asked him why he was locked up in Administrative Segregation, he told me it was because the white guards were afraid of him.

"Why are they afraid of you?," I asked.

"Because I am an African Chief, and they know that I can call my tribe together on the yard and tell them to kill any guard who disrespects me."

Mr. P.'s security file contains a note that he spit at a guard a month prior to our interview and received a write-up for assaulting an officer. When I ask him about the incident, he tells me,"I didn't assault anyone, he assaulted me." I ask why a guard would single him out for abuse, and he responds: "It's only the white guards. They're afraid of my power. They say I'm in a gang, but I'm not. I'm in a tribe. I'm the chief of an African tribe. White men have been coming to Africa and stealing my people and making them into slaves. I came here to take them back. The guards know that. There's one black guard on the night shift. He knows I'm a chief, so he leaves me alone. The white guards are out to get me. They're always picking fights with me, then they say I assaulted them."

O'Neill Stough, a white prisoner who is very perceptive when it comes to race relations in correctional settings, comments that although black prisoners are definitely treated more harshly, all prisoners suffer on account of unfair and abusive practices on the part of correctional staff:

> Years of seeing your fellow man brutalized and harassed by . . . [prison guards], and prisoner-on-prisoner beatings, threats, killing, rapes, etc., takes its toll on your psyche. You begin to question the authority which allows such inhumanity, and soon, to question society itself, which seems to condone such abuses by its silence. A festering anger begins to grow, a resentment for the hypocrisy of a system that purports to represent justice, but in practice dispenses gross injustice on a daily basis.

## Access to Mental Health Treatment

When mental health services are provided in an interracial setting, and especially when the provider is white and the prisoner/patient is a person of color, the clinical situation is complicated. Misunderstandings and miscommunications abound.

One simple example: The difference between "paranoia" and "protective awareness" has much to do with the color of one's skin. The fact that a white clinician has trouble understanding why a black prisoner feels he is being persecuted has something to do with the fact that the black man has been frequently stopped, frisked, and harassed by police on the outside and guards inside, whereas the white clinician relies on the police in both settings to protect him. Often the white clinician assumes the black prisoner is paranoid about the extent of racism in the prison even though the black man is merely exhibiting a protective awareness about a reality that is more dangerous than the white man will ever know.

Racial discrimination is often involved in the decision to punish an individual or send him to see a therapist. School teachers suspend impoverished black children for the same unacceptable behaviors that trigger a referral to see a therapist when the culprit is a middle-class white child. Similarly, when police are called to control an angry black male who is acting bizarrely, they are very likely to arrest him without considering very seriously the possibility he might be suffering from a mental disorder. The same police officers, when called to a middle-class home to contain a disruptive male, are much more likely to cart him off to a psychiatric hospital.

Poor people of color tend to have very little access to talking therapy, and when their psychiatric disabilities grow to emergency proportions, they tend to be medicated in psychiatric emergency rooms or admitted to a hospital for a very brief stay. In contrast, affluent white people are more likely to seek out and be able to afford some kind of psychotherapy when crises arise, even if they are prescribed medications at the same time. In other words, there is a double standard in the provision of mental health services in the community: Talking therapy is reserved for the affluent, pills and involuntary hospitalization for the poor.

In prison, the same double standard exists. Access to treatment depends on the staff recognizing that problematic behaviors such as self-imposed isolation in a cell, rule-breaking, and fighting are due, to a significant extent, to mental illness. Staff also need to conclude that the problematic behaviors are not merely manipulative. I have found that guards tend to be more empathic with prisoners who share their cultural background. For instance, in several prisons I have toured, prisoners of color complain that the guards give white prisoners the equivalent of a slap on the wrist for the same offenses that land black prisoners in solitary confinement for months. Or prisoners of color tell me that a mentally disordered white prisoner is sent to a relatively comfortable mental health program because the staff decide his rule violations result from his mental disorder, whereas a black or Latino prisoner who is just as disturbed and breaks an equivalent rule is sent to lock-up. Indeed, white prisoners are overrepresented in most prison mental health programs, whereas people of color, including prisoners suffering from severe mental disorders, are grossly overrepresented in the lock-up units.

Even inside the lock-up units, prisoners of color who exhibit signs of severe mental illness are more likely to be disciplined than they are to be treated adequately. For example:

> Vinson, an African-American man, was confined in the Security Housing Unit at Pelican Bay State Prison in California. He displayed significant psychiatric symptomatology. Notes in his clinical chart indicate that several clinicians suspected he was suffering from a psychotic condition replete with hallucinations and delusions, but each added that he might be malingering. They were "observing" him and considering a transfer to a psychiatric inpatient unit in another prison. But there was no follow-up to any of these notes, and Vinson was left in solitary confinement, where he regressed and began to smear himself with feces.
>
> On April 22, 1992, the white guards on duty noticed the odor and, without bothering to speak to a psychiatrist about possible alternative interventions, decided to intervene forcefully. First they ordered him to take a bath. When he refused, they did a cell extraction, escorted him to the infirmary in chains and forced him into a bathtub filled with scalding hot water and at least one corrosive chemical substance. Several correctional officers pushed his head under the water. He screamed in pain. They ignored his distress. Then he fainted and had to be removed from the bath.
>
> When Vinson emerged from this forced dunking, it was noted that the skin was peeling off his back, legs, and buttocks. He suffered severe, third-degree burns that required skin grafts over a significant portion of his body. And still there were ugly scars. He won a personal lawsuit, his case was brought to the attention of the court in several large class action lawsuits, and Amnesty International labeled the incident "torture."

I interviewed Vinson six months after this incident. He told me that he believes that he was the victim of racism. He stressed that he was a grown man and did not need to be given a bath. He claimed that a bottle of some toxic liquid substance and a cup of powdered substance were poured into the hot water in the tub. He protested the brutal dunking, but the officers proceeded to push his head under the water. Even though he was in great pain he did not scream because he did not want them to think he was a "pussy."

Racial discrimination in the provision of mental health treatment is not limited to prisoners suffering from serious mental disorders. White drug offenders are more likely to receive treatment, in the community as well as in correctional facilities, whereas people of color are more likely to be incarcerated for their drug offenses and, once in prison, less likely than whites to be included in drug rehabilitation programs. A recent California study showed that two-thirds of prison drug treatment slots went to whites even though 70 percent of inmates sentenced for drug offenses were African American. A study in New York revealed the same pattern.

Racial divides and overt racism are omnipresent in prison. Even if a prisoner knows he is prone to emotional dyscontrol whenever he gets into an interracial altercation, it is not possible for him to avoid potentially hazardous situations. Prisoners of color are doubly affected by racial discrimination behind bars. Racism plays a big part in the evolution and exacerbation of their psychiatric symptomatology, and they are more likely than whites to be denied adequate mental health services.

---

Racism is not the only form of domination in correctional settings. In the next chapter I examine ways women prisoners suffer when their special needs are ignored and they become victims of sexual harassment.

# 5

# Special Problems for Women

Gender differences matter quite a lot behind bars. Women suffer different traumas than do men before going to prison. They are convicted of crimes for different reasons, their needs and the problems they have coping with life in prison are very distinct, and their emotional reactions are quite different. If we are to understand the emotional difficulties that plague many prisoners, we have to consider their backgrounds, the obstacles they face as mothers in prison, other special needs they have as women, the kind of harsh conditions and discipline they are forced to endure, and the sexual harassment that goes along with being a women prisoner.

Men's and women's prisons are equivalent in many ways. Racism is as big a problem in women's facilities as it is in men's—over 50 percent of women incarcerated in state and federal prisons are people of color, and nineteen of the forty-three women on death row in 1993 were African American or Latina. Punitive segregation and solitary confinement units cause the same pain and suffering to both genders, and a lack of meaningful education and rehabilitation programs makes it difficult for all prisoners to succeed in the community after their release.

But there are also striking contrasts between women and men behind bars, beginning with the reasons they are incarcerated. A large majority of the crimes that land women in prison are nonviolent—80 percent in some states—and 60 percent are drug-related. Women are much less likely to commit assault and homicide than men. Men who commit violent crimes are more likely to assault a stranger, often in the course of a robbery, whereas women are much more likely to assault someone they know.

Fifty-one percent of homicide convictions for women involve murdering a partner, usually after he has beaten or raped her, and half of the forty-five women on Death Row nationwide in 1993 were there for the murder of an abusive spouse or lover. Approximately 80 percent of women behind bars have been the victims of domestic violence and physical or sexual abuse at some time prior to their conviction. Most women imprisoned for killing an abusive partner are first-time offenders. And women who have been convicted of a violent offense are much less likely than men convicted of equivalent offenses to be re-arrested for a violent offense after their release.

Studies show there is a high incidence of depression in women prisoners—higher than in men. Perhaps it is merely a matter of men acting out their emotional turmoil in aggressive acts that draw a lot of attention, whereas women suffer their depressions silently. But we also know that the experiences that make women prisoners a unique group—their long history of abuse, their deep commitment to mothering, difficulty in maintaining self-esteem for an entire prison term filled with harsh treatment and sexual harassment—are also serious risk factors for depression and other forms of emotional distress. And once women prisoners develop a significant emotional disorder, the inadequacies of correctional mental health services cause them undue hardship.

## Gender Differences

In many cases, the gender differences that exist on the outside are exaggerated in prison. For instance, a large proportion of female felons are single mothers and serve as the primary parent in their households. When they go to prison, separation from their children becomes excruciatingly painful.

Another problem is the inattention and even abuse women receive in relation to their special needs. They cannot wear the clothes they would like. They cannot have the privacy they'd been accustomed to. They cannot have quality contact with the people they care most about. These and other losses wear on them. They feel lonely. They get sad, or angry, or they cut off all their emotions and fall into depression.

Since prison rules and classification systems were designed with men in mind, their application in women's facilities can have very adverse ramifications. There are rules and procedures in prison for just about everything, including where a prisoner can walk and how much time she can spend alone. There are a rapidly growing number of rules about the length of a prisoner's hair, the piercings and tattoos that are permissible, and the limits on a prisoner's possessions. The higher a prisoner's security classification level, the more restrictions there are. But when the male-oriented rules and classification system are applied to women, causing their special needs to be ignored and excessive force to be used to control them, they suffer severe and unnecessary hardship. If a woman is prone to emotional disorder of any kind, the suffering tends to make her condition worse.

## Women and Children

Eighty percent of women prisoners have children. Seventy percent of prisoners who have children are single mothers, and 85 percent had custody of their children prior to incarceration. I am told that it's extremely difficult and painful to be a mother in prison. As a man, I can only know that from listening to women's stories, or by imagining what a hellish place prisons must be for mothers. How can they stay connected to their children while they are locked up? How can they keep them out of harm's way? Visiting privileges take on a special meaning when visits are the only time a mother can see her children. And mother's mental stability depends on her knowing her children are receiving good care.

Six percent of women convicts are pregnant when they enter prison and give birth inside. Prenatal care in most women's prisons is very inadequate. A recent poll of state prisons for women found that 58 percent of them provided pregnant women with the same food that all prisoners receive, and that tends not to be a very healthy prenatal diet. And there is very little psychotherapy available for women who have lost babies or had abortions inside.

Women who give birth inside prison are usually pressured to give the babies up for adoption. Except in the relatively few facilities where women are permitted to keep their newborn babies with them, mothers are forced to give them up at birth. If they aren't lucky enough to find a relative who will agree to raise their child, they are forced to give the infant up for blind adoption. There may not be a written policy requiring women prisoners to give up their parental rights, but when the staff put pressure on a pregnant woman to give up custody by arguing that the child will be much better off in another family, and the pregnant prisoner is already suffering from shame, remorse, and low self-esteem, she feels coerced into complying and signing over custody.

There is some variation between the states in regard to prisoners who give birth inside the institutions. For instance, the Bedford Hills Correctional Facility in New York contains a nursery program that provides some women who give birth inside the opportunity to keep their babies in the prison for up to a year to allow for mother-child bonding. But in most states, even where there is a baby nursery and a program that permits mothers to have significant contact with their young children, the shortage of spaces and requirements for admission to the program make it impossible for a large proportion of mothers to receive the benefit. For instance, in California there are fewer than a dozen spots for prisoner/mothers in special residential units where they can keep their very young children with them and receive training in mothering, and any prisoner who is not classified a very low security risk is barred from participating in the program.

For a woman who already has children when she enters prison, the biggest problem is finding a way to maintain her family's integrity while she is behind bars. If the father is present, then she worries about maintaining their marital relationship. Perhaps she worries that he will stray, or drink and abuse the children. For single mothers, there is the issue of losing the children altogether. Perhaps a relative has taken them while the mother is behind bars, or they might have become wards of the court. Will they be alright? Will they ever be back with their mother? These questions plague mothers throughout their terms. If the answers are gloomy, there is likely to be shame, depression, and self-destruction.

Mothers in prison are less likely to be visited by their children than are fathers. This is because the mother who is free typically brings the children to see the father when he is imprisoned, but when she goes to prison, especially if she is a single mother, she loses custody while inside, and there may be no one to bring her children to see her. There are also structural problems that make it difficult for women to stay in touch with their children. There are fewer women's prisons than men's, so they tend to be situated further from the average inmate's home. Some states and the federal system transfer women out of state because of a shortage of women's beds. One state might "rent" space in another state's prisons. Of course, this makes it more difficult to keep in touch with loved ones.

Many women suffer from depression related to losing their children and the break-up of their families. Former prisoner Geraldine explains:

> Even though I did well in prison, I would have these periods every six months or every nine months when I would hit this bottom. I would get so severely depressed about not seeing my son and my family, about just wanting to be free. After a while, you cannot take the confinement

> any more. You're so totally secluded from everything. I was fortunate. My family came to visit me three or four times a year. My older sister and her husband raised my son from the time he was two, and the blessing was that they always allowed me to be a part of his life. I had seen women in prison break up telephone receivers because they would tell them, no, you can't talk to your child, we don't want you in her life any more.

But treatment for this kind of depression behind bars is far from adequate. As in men's prisons, women who suffer from depression may be given psychotropic medications, but they receive very little quality counseling or therapy. In a clinical setting outside of prison, for instance in a psychiatric hospital or residential program, outreach by a social worker is a critical part of a depressed woman's mental health treatment. The assumption is that the woman's depression has much to do with her role as a mother, and if she is unable to have much contact with her children, at least a social worker can stay in touch with them and keep the mother posted about how they are doing. But in prison, outreach by social workers is a very rare event. Even when the termination of a pregnancy or loss of a child is at stake, and some kind of talking interaction with a competent professional is very much needed, little help is available.

## Appearance, Individuality, and Self-Esteem

My recent experience as an expert witness in a prison lawsuit provided some insight into the special needs and problems of women prisoners. I testified as a psychiatric expert about the possible ill effects on prisoners' mental health of a proposed new policy directive requiring Michigan prisoners to wear uniforms and give up most of their possessions. *Cain* v. *Michigan Department of Corrections (MDOC)*, a class action lawsuit brought on behalf of 41,000 male and 2,000 female state prisoners, has been ongoing for ten years. The effect of the legal action so far has been to halt the state from fully implementing the new policy directive. The prisoners claim the state-issue uniforms are totally inadequate for the Michigan climate. And if the new policy directive were to go into effect, the prisoners would have to give up all possessions that can't fit into a duffel bag (prisoners housed in maximum and supermaximum security facilities) or a duffel bag and small footlocker (prisoners housed in minimum and medium security prisons).

The new policy would restrict prisoners' possessions in other ways. For instance, all possessions would have to be purchased new from a mail order catalogue of the single company approved by the department of corrections for supplying prisoners. The prisoners would no longer be able to have their families send them clothes and other items, and they would be unable to purchase used clothing or have their families shop around for less expensive items. In addition, if a prisoner were to be transferred to a higher security classification, for instance to a lock-up unit, and eventually win an appeal of the decision and be sent back to a lower-level institution, she would have lost all of her possessions in the process and have to purchase all new things. Obviously, this policy would create immense hardship for prisoners of limited means.

In preparation for my testimony in *Cain* v. *MDOC*, I asked the eight prisoners who are acting *in pro se* (as their own attorneys—in collaboration with attorneys assigned to the case) to send a questionnaire to a number of prisoners so that I could determine what they believe they would have to give up were the new policy to be enacted, and how that would affect them. The questionnaire was sent to seventy male prisoners in twenty-four institutions and twenty female prisoners in three institutions. The prisoners were so excited about the prospect of telling their stories that I received responses from 461 men and 260 women. Many respondents simply looked over the shoulders of those who possessed copies of the questionnaire and wrote out their numbered answers on blank sheets of paper. What a testimonial to the desire of silenced voices to be heard!

The prisoners' responses to the questionnaire provide an opportunity to understand some of their concerns as well as the potential impact of the new policy on prisoners' mental health. Both men and women predicted they would have to give up approximately the same possessions, including legal materials, photos in frames and albums, musical and educational tapes and records, athletic equipment such as handballs and weight-lifting belts, musical instruments, art and hobbycraft supplies, religious books and artifacts, soap and toilet items, and a large amount of clothing such as winter coats, bathrobes, athletic shoes and outfits, and items with sentimental value.

There were sharp gender differences in prisoners' responses to questions about how they would feel were they to lose most of their possessions and have to wear uniforms. For the men, the most frequent responses involve anger, a need for retaliation, and the assumption the prison would be much less safe since all the men would feel the same way. For the women, the most frequent responses involve diminished self-worth, loss of identity, depression, shame, isolation, and feeling violated. The gender differences are not surprising. It is well known that men tend to respond to trauma by acting out aggressively whereas women are more likely to turn their negative feelings inward and become depressed.

The women all share certain core concerns about clothing, make-up, and appearance. While the men complain they will not be able to participate in athletic endeavors and strenuous work because they will only have one set of clothes while the other set is in the laundry, the women express more specific concerns, usually related to self-esteem and a sense of degradation. One woman writes:

> One could argue that self-esteem and identity are not based upon dress and appearance. I categorically deny that. My recent and hard-fought rise in self-esteem shows that I have been tending to my appearance—in the clothing I choose, the make-up I choose to wear, in my

> overall attitude about myself. To lose the ability to care for myself and nurture myself in this most basic of ways would be devastating.

A forty-five-year-old woman serving a six- to twenty-eight-year sentence in a minimum security prison writes that having her possessions taken from her would make her feel: "Angry, dehumanized, depressed, disconnected, unlovable, unwanted, defeminized, and deindividualized." Her response to a question about giving up her personal clothing and having to wear uniforms: "Traumatic, upsetting. I have nothing else left in my life that I can call my own. Everything I knew and loved is gone—my family, my home, my freedom. The only things I have in my life right now and for the next several years that belong to me are a few measly pieces of comfortable, much-worn clothing. It is really my only tie with humanity that keeps this whole terrible environment from overwhelming me!"

Histories of abuse prior to incarceration show up frequently, even though no question addressed the issue of domestic violence. For instance, responding to the same question about giving up personal clothing, a forty-seven-year-old woman with two children who is serving a life sentence for killing her abusive husband writes:

> During my seventeen-year marriage, I developed a psychological profile similar to that of a prisoner of war. I went through many things which lowered my self-esteem including being told what to wear, when to wear it, and how to wear it. During my incarceration, I have accomplished many things, one of which is I feel a certain independence at being able to make decisions for myself, including what to put on every day. If my clothes are taken from me, I fear emotionally, mentally, and psychologically I will be going backward, again feeling like I did all those years ago in my abusive marriage. If this

> backward movement within myself takes place, I question whether I will again harm someone I may conceive as an abuser.

The same woman writes in response to a different question:

> I am unable to obtain brassieres in my size and if I do happen to get any, they do not give me the support needed for as well endowed as I am. Other females are getting used bras [prison issue uniforms would include undergarments, the plan being for prisoners to exchange their dirty clothes for a clean but not personal set from the laundry] which tells me the department of corrections cannot properly dress females. The blues that are issued have holes and tears in them and are made for men. This means they are not fitted properly for a woman.

A forty-nine-year-old woman with three children writes:

> The new policy allows for only one pair of shoes. . . . No dresses or skirts creates another dilemma in my life. When I attend church I am forced to wear pants because I don't have any shoes to wear with a dress. From an early age, I was taught women wear dresses to church. I feel a certain amount of embarrassment and guilt attending church in pants.
>
> My identity is torn apart when I am forced to wear men's clothing. I am a lady and I want to dress like one. Shirts and pants issued by the state are male. The new property policy states I can only have a male white T-shirt. When women wear them, the bra is clearly seen. This facility is run predominantly by males. Therefore, I feel visually raped every time I must wear the white T-

> shirt. Furthermore, since I have a full chest, I feel very self-conscious knowing that my bra is exposed. In my family, my sisters and I were taught it is degrading to expose our undergarments.

When I took the stand in *Cain* v. *MDOC*, I read some of the prisoners' responses and pointed out ways their narrative comments mirrored what we know from clinical research. For instance, when women's needs are systematically ignored they are likely to feel abused and oppressed, and the result can be emotional breakdown.

At this writing, the Cain case is still in trial, and although the judge is permitting the state to implement parts of the draconian policy, he is also granting the prisoners some relief in relation to specific issues. For example, he has ordered the state to permit the prisoners to retain their overcoats and gloves. However, in several other states, prisoners are being forced to buy all their gear from approved catalogues, cut their hair short, and forego gifts from home, and women are being forced to wear men's clothing and used bras.

## Classification and Discipline

Women's prisons are modeled after men's. It would be more accurate to say that women's prisons are an afterthought. Until well into the twentieth century, many women's prisons were merely partitioned-off sections of men's facilities. The same rules that applied to the men were enforced with women. That tendency is still in place today. For instance, even though there is much less violence and almost no escape attempts at women's prisons, women who break rules are placed in lock-up units that were designed for very violent men. I do not support the use of excessive force and isolation with the men. But certainly, when equivalent force is used against women, something is terribly wrong.

In prison, order is maintained by a classification system and clear disciplinary procedures. The same "points" that determine men's security classification levels are usually applied to women prisoners. For example, very long sentences are meted out today for victimless crimes such as drug possession. This means that a woman who has a previous criminal record—and for many women this means minor offenses such as check-forgery, shoplifting, and vagrancy—and a long sentence to serve for a drug offense could be sent to a high-security prison even though she has never been convicted of a violent offense, has never broken the rules in a correctional setting, and poses virtually no escape risk. When she is sent to the high-security facility, where conditions are harsher, she is moved further from home and her children and forced to be more idle and isolated than she would be at a lower security level. The harshness, relative lack of meaningful activities, and enhanced isolation can have devastating psychiatric effects.

Classification systems can put women at a disadvantage in many other ways. The smaller scale of women's prison systems means that fewer services and programs, including mental health services, are available in each prison, and the women have to be moved around more than the men when they are assigned to a different security level or a different program. For instance, in Michigan's state prisons, mental health services for men are available at all classification levels, but the only significant mental health services available for women prisoners are situated in level 4 and 5 maximum security institutions. This means that a woman prisoner in a minimum security facility who suffers an emotional breakdown must be transferred to a much higher security level if she is to undergo psychiatric treatment. In the process, even though she has not done anything wrong, she will lose her job as well as many privileges.

In terms of disciplinary procedures, there tend to be more rules for women, and the rules tend to be pettier. For instance, there are often rules about keeping one's cell clean or acting appropriately at the dinner table. It's as though the women are being closely monitored for deviance from acceptable feminine behavior. Women report the staff infantilize them, calling them "bad girls," or just "girls." Women prisoners tend to receive disciplinary citations more often than men. But more of the women's citations are for minor rule infractions, things for which the men would not be cited, whereas the men's citations tend to be for more serious offenses. In contrast to the men, who are angered by this kind of close surveillance and pettiness, women prisoners who are subjected to these kinds of disciplinary procedures tend to experience intensified shame, anxiety, and depression.

Even though most of the women in high-security prisons have broken many minor rules but have never been written up for very violent acts or serious infractions, there are supermaximum control units for women in many states. As in men's facilities, as soon as supermaximum control units are established, mentally disordered prisoners find their way into them, and the isolation and idleness cause their conditions to deteriorate further.

Some state departments of corrections even conduct cell extractions in the maximum and supermaximum security units for women. Imagine five large guards barging into a cell behind a lexan shield to subdue one woman! The very thought of this kind of brutality makes many women prisoners fear for their lives. Anxiety and panic disorder are not included on the list of "major mental disorders," but I have encountered quite a few women suffering from severe generalized anxiety and panic attacks in women's maximum and supermaximum security units. Of course, physical brutality is not the only abuse the women fear.

## Sexual Harassment

When male staff are put in charge of women prisoners, and the architecture and policies of the prisons permit or require staff to observe and intrude constantly into the daily activities of their wards, there are daily incidents of sexual harassment. And in the prisons where sexual harassment is the most blatant, there is little or no recourse for the victimized prisoners.

Since many of the women have histories that include childhood physical and sexual abuse and some degree of domestic violence or rape as adults, the awful incidents that occur during a prison term serve as replays of earlier traumas and set off powerful emotional reactions. In women who are prone to psychosis, the reaction can be a complete breakdown. In women who suffer from posttraumatic stress disorder, the reaction is usually intensified flashbacks and nightmares. Women who tend to fall into depression report that traumatic prison experiences lead to more serious depressions.

## Panopticism in Women's Institutions

There is a trend in modern prison design toward total observation of prisoners. Control booths placed in the center of cell pods make it possible for the officer in the booth to directly observe all of the prisoners and control their movements by opening and shutting doors via remote control. This architectural innovation is modeled on Jeremy Bentham's "panopticon," a prison designed to leave prisoners no place to hide from surveillance. Bentham believed the prisoner who is forced to undergo total surveillance will eventually give up her devious, criminal ways and become the kind of citizen who has nothing to hide. Michel Foucault believed the most important effect of "panopticism" was to induce in the prisoner "a state of conscious and permanent visibility that assures the automatic functioning of power." There are some short-term security advantages to this design. A relatively small number of guards are able to maintain order in a large unit. The danger is that the total lack of privacy will cause severe hardship for prisoners.

An aggravating factor in prisons for women is the presence of male guards. Up until the 1960s, male guards were in the minority in most women's facilities and were not permitted unsupervised contact with inmates. But following the Civil Rights Act of 1964 and other equal employment legislation, the proportion of male staff began to rise. Today, the ratio of men to women corrections officers in women's prisons is at least two to one.

I have discovered many very paranoid prisoners in male units designed for direct and total observation, and they tell me their decompensation began with the uncomfortable feeling they were being watched all the time. In women's prisons, this kind of panopticism means that male guards are often in a position to view women in states of undress, on the toilet, and in the shower. Where there is malevolence on the part of the guards, this is a set-up for sexual harassment. But even when no malevolence is intended, and especially when the women have had the experience earlier in their lives of males violating their boundaries in traumatic ways, the lack of privacy can be humiliating and shame-inducing.

Male prisoners tend not to complain about the presence of female security officers on their tiers. They might mention that the presence of women makes them a little self-conscious using the toilet, but they do not report women officers gawking at them when they are exposed. In fact, where I have seen men taking showers while women officers are on duty, male officers are assigned to supervise the showers, or the male prisoners are asked to wear robes while walking to and from the shower area. It is true that male prisoners sometimes purposely strip and expose themselves in front of female staff. I have heard of cases where a male prisoner, usually one suffering from a serious mental disorder, masturbates just as a female officer is due to pass by his cell. But in most prisons, exhibitionistic and abusive behavior on the part of male prisoners is severely punished.

Much less care is taken to respect the modesty of female prisoners when male guards are on duty, and there is a much greater tendency for male guards to take advantage of their power and harass the women. A woman in a maximum security prison informs me that there is usually one male guard on duty on her tier during the evening shift. The women are locked in for the evening and he patrols the "freeway" that runs along the front of their "houses" or cells. "It seems like every time you use the toilet or begin to undress for bed, he's standing there in front of your cell gawking at you.

Sometimes he rubs his crotch and makes some crude comment about wanting to do something to you or have you do something to him. It's so disgusting, and there's nothing you can do about it because he's totally in charge."

Not all male staff harass female prisoners. Many women report that the kindness of certain male guards has been one of the main supports for them while serving their time. But there are structural aspects of the program in women's prisons that make sexual harassment an everyday occurrence, even when male staff do not mean to be abusive. Besides the trend toward total visibility, there are the humiliating search procedures. Of course, when a male guard exploits his authority and sexually harasses a female prisoner, there is inexcusable malice—an all too common occurrence according to reports I hear from women prisoners. The policies for searching prisoners—the arbitrariness of the searches, the ease with which staff can use such searches as a way to punish and harass prisoners they consider troublemakers, the lack of recourse for prisoners who feel they are being treated unfairly—set up a situation that permits sexual harassment and rape to occur and go undetected.

Prisoners have to submit to body searches at any time of day or night. Officers can order a prisoner to strip and submit to a body cavity probe on the spot. Women in maximum security units are made to kneel on all fours for vaginal and rectal searches. Obviously, when the search is conducted by male officers, there is a high likelihood of abuse. If they choose to rub a woman's breast in the process, or spend extra time examining her crotch or exploring a body cavity, there is little the female prisoner can do without risking a write-up for refusing to follow an order or disrespecting an officer.

Strip searches and probes of body cavities in women's prisons, especially when men are nearby or involved in the procedure, create an ambience of intimidation and disrespect that implies official toleration of sexual harassment and rape. A certain number of security measures are necessary in a prison, but I have heard from a large number of staff and prisoners alike that most strip searches and probes of body cavities could be discontinued with no additional threat to institutional security.

Since a large proportion of women prisoners have suffered physical and sexual abuse in the past, they are all too familiar with the kind of patronizing, demeaning, and frequently abusive treatment they receive as prisoners. And they have learned from cruel experience that resisting very often leads to further abuse. Often it's a case of repeatedly traumatized women not standing up for their rights because they are trying very hard to fit in and feel like they belong for a change. But the sense of fitting in is too often purchased at the cost of continuing shame, self-hatred, and depression.

An African-American woman in her early thirties who is serving a second term for drug possession in a maximum security women's prison tells me she graduated from college and supported herself and her baby before she was convicted and sent to this prison:

> But in here they infantilize you in every way they can, demeaning you, treating you like a bad girl, until you don't have any will left to fight them, you forget how to think for yourself, you just go along and say "OK, I guess I am just what you say I am," and then, since you're so totally dependent on them, even to bring you a tampon during your monthly, you hope that since you've confessed to being bad and you're willing to play their little games, they will at least take care of you and not let you die of neglect.

## Mental Health Issues

Although the prevalence of serious mental disorders is approximately the same for women and men, there are some differences. For instance, epidemiological research shows that women in the community suffer slightly more often than men from depressions serious enough to warrant professional intervention, and a larger proportion of women suffer psychiatric symptoms secondary to sexual and physical abuse. It's difficult to arrive at precise prevalence rates because women are much more likely than men to seek professional help. In prison, the gender differences are in the same direction but even more pronounced, and it is even more difficult to determine prevalence rates for women because of severe underdiagnosis.

## Depression

It is quite obvious that women in prison are more prone to depression whereas men are more prone to the kind of angry outbursts that land them in lock-up situations. Of course, there are exceptions in both directions. I mention in Chapter Two that a significant number of men withdraw into their cells for protection and then experience depression. And some women get angry and strike out. But since women are taught from an early age to turn their dissatisfactions and resentments inward and stay out of trouble, far fewer act out violently in prison and they are more likely than male prisoners to suffer in silence and not even request mental health treatment.

If we were to explore the reasons for a woman prisoner's depression and anxiety, there would be many things to consider. Is she still suffering aftereffects of the sexual abuse she suffered as a preteen? Did the drugs she resorted to in hopes of forgetting cause permanent brain damage and a lasting mental disorder? Did all those beatings at her partner's hands cause a chronic posttraumatic stress disorder that only looks like a depression? Is she thinking obsessively about the terrible person she is for doing the crime and winding up in prison and far from her children? Is she worrying she will never be able to forgive herself if anything bad happens to them?

The prevalence of posttraumatic stress disorder among women prisoners is certainly higher than in the community. A lifetime of sexual and physical abuse causes severe emotional distress. But a large group of women who suffer posttraumatic symptoms are misdiagnosed by mental health staff as suffering from "hysterical personality" or "borderline personality disorder." When a woman is assertive, upset, emotionally expressive, and dissatisfied with the services she is receiving, the mental health staff are likely to dismiss her as "just another borderline trying to manipulate us to get more attention." Since the overextended mental health staff in correctional settings are advised to avoid having their time monopolized by manipulative prisoners with personality disorders, and to treat only "major mental illnesses," the diagnosis of hysterical personality or borderline personality disorder makes it very unlikely that a woman will receive any significant mental health services. In other words, the diagnosis is a wastebasket category for traumatized and undertreated women in prison.

## Complex PTSD

Psychiatrist Judith Herman, after treating a large number of women survivors of repeated sexual and physical abuse, has come to the conclusion that they are very often diagnosed with a personality disorder while the underlying posttraumatic picture is missed. Whether they are identified as "masochistic," "histrionic," "self-defeating personality," "somatization disorder," or "borderline," there is a tendency for care-providers to blame the victim of repetitive abuse as if her weak personality or flawed character was the cause of the traumas she was forced to endure. Herman proposes a new diagnostic category for survivors of repetitive abuse whose chronic symptoms include severe depression, emotional lability, multiple somatic complaints, and smoldering anger: complex posttraumatic stress disorder. Once it's recognized that accumulated traumas from the past are the cause of current emotional distress, it's possible to provide an opportunity for these women to establish a modicum of safety in their current lives and talk through the past traumas on their way to recovery.

Posttraumatic stress disorders are often complicated by substance abuse, and in a large proportion of cases, mental health practitioners identify the substance abuse as the single psychiatric problem and miss the earlier and ongoing traumas. Many women prisoners resorted to drugs and alcohol in large part to block out flashbacks and numb the pain. And unless the underlying traumatic memories are brought to the surface and worked through, there is a great likelihood that these women will return to using drugs and alcohol after they are released from prison.

Likewise, interviews with sex workers and women who are repeatedly battered very frequently turn up a history of repetitive sexual and physical abuse since early childhood. Unless the history of abuse is uncovered, it is quite likely that once these women are released they will return to the kinds of abusive relationships that led to their law-breaking and imprisonment.

## The Absence of Treatment

Many prison mental health services are limited to a psychiatrist who visits periodically to prescribe strong psychotropic medications. There may also be a few psychologists who spend most of their time administering psychological tests for courts and the parole board, and nurses who barely have time to evaluate emergency cases and pass out pills. But there is no place for a woman who has been massively traumatized and feels depressed or angry to talk through her traumatic memories in a therapeutic setting.

We know what people who suffer from the aftereffects of severe and repeated trauma need in terms of treatment. Mainly, women who have been traumatized need a safe place to talk. Medications can be useful as adjuncts to talking therapy—for instance, in the treatment of severe anxiety, depression, and psychotic reactions—but the prescription of medications for women suffering from post-traumatic stress disorder can be quite tricky. If tranquilizers are prescribed to keep the trauma survivor from experiencing any significant degree of anxiety or rage, for example, the survivor might begin to feel that her emotional reactions are suspect, bringing the active grieving process to a halt and trapping the survivor in a chronic numbing process. Too often the pattern leads to chronic depression and long-term reliance on tranquilizing medications to ward off intrusive symptoms.

Alternatively, antidepressant medications can be appropriately prescribed for a woman who feels numb and appears depressed. But prescribing antidepressants in the absence of counseling sessions runs the risk of too rapidly arousing the survivor from a state of numbed depression only to be terrorized anew by awful memories, flashbacks, and nightmares. There is a heightened risk of suicide at such moments. We can only guess how many suicides among women prisoners taking antidepressants fit this tragic picture. I will not go into any greater detail here about the medication management of PTSD, except to say it is a complicated endeavor.

The key question is whether medications are being prescribed as an adjunct to the critical therapeutic task of talking through the trauma, or as a substitute for the opportunity to talk and work through the emotional crisis. In many women's prisons, because the mental health services are inadequate and the harried mental health staff tend to dismiss many survivors of chronic abuse as manipulators or "borderlines," a large number of women are ignored and left to their own devices, or prescribed medications alone when they complain of unbearable emotional symptoms.

In most women's institutions, just as in men's, there is little or no group therapy. There is very little help with substance abuse problems. And women who have been raped and brutalized are unable to see a therapist of any kind, unless they suffer a total breakdown and get sent to an inpatient psychiatric facility. Even there, they may stay for a short period only and are unlikely to have much opportunity to talk to a therapist who could help them recover and heal.

Not all or even a majority of women prisoners suffer from emotional disorders. I am always impressed by the number of prisoners who are able to cope with the reality of imprisonment and set about preparing themselves for their eventual release and reunion with family. Not all women prisoners were abused as children and beaten as adults. And not all abused women have difficulty coping emotionally. I am amazed at the resilience exhibited by women and men who have survived massive and repeated traumas in their lives and continue to carry on remarkably satisfying lives, even in prison. But a significant number of women prisoners do experience emotional reactions that overwhelm their capacity to cope, and they need mental health treatment.

## Preparation for Going Straight

I am sad to report that in many women's prisons an attitude of condescension is reflected in the design of mental health treatment programs and nonclinical rehabilitation programs. As a rule, less money and effort are spent on designing and running rehabilitation programs for women compared to men. But even where there are programs, they are not as effective as they need to be if the women are to succeed after they are released. Women prisoners are given menial jobs, and if training is available in prison, it is usually aimed at low-income positions such as food preparation, cleaning, and secretarial work. Many very bright women prisoners are given little or no opportunity to pursue an education or meaningful and somewhat challenging training. And very few women are provided the kind of psychiatric and substance abuse treatment that they need to work through earlier traumas and continuing problems with self-esteem.

Even the women who are lucky enough to maintain a meaningful job or training slot inside prison will be released with very little in the way of postrelease support programs. Ex-prisoners report that it is practically impossible to find work in the community after they are released, and there are no social service workers available to help them reunite with and support their families. Of course, this lack of postrelease support makes a return to drugs and crime all the more likely. It also explains why so many women who have served time in prison suffer from chronic depression.

---

There is a price the women and the society to which they return pay for the shortcomings of their prison experience. A forty-nine-year-old woman in the final third of her fifteen-year sentence for second degree murder confides: "I'm beginning to think about leaving this place. I worry about the reentry, about being able to make choices again, open doors for myself, picking out what I want to eat for the first time in ten years."

Unfortunately, in all too many cases, what is done to women behind bars—including the humiliation, sexual harassment, separation from their loved ones, lack of meaningful rehabilitation, and the patronizing attitude of the staff—makes their postrelease adjustment very difficult indeed. But I don't want to give the impression that all or even most women felons are victims who fall into passivity and depression. The things that are done to women prisoners tend to cause depression and other forms of emotional disturbance. I always find it amazing how many women maintain their mental stability and function very well, for instance as mothers, even while doing time under very harsh and oppressive conditions.

---

Rape is one of the most horrifying abuses that occur on a regular basis in both women's and men's prisons. When rape occurs in women's prisons, it is usually committed by male staff. For women and men alike the emotional repercussions can be devastating, and this is the topic of the next chapter.

# 6

# Rape and Posttraumatic Stress Disorder

The incidence of rape behind bars is high. No precise figure is available because so many incidents go unreported. Among men, at least a quarter in correctional facilities say they have been pressured for sex. The Federal Bureau of Prisons estimates that between 9 and 20 percent of male prisoners become victims of sexual assault during their prison terms. This is probably a very conservative estimate. And the incidence would be much higher if the figure included all the cases in which an inmate "agrees" to participate in sexual acts only because he fears that refusal will lead to a beating and rape. Many seemingly "voluntary" sexual acts are actually coerced.

It is even more difficult to estimate the incidence of rape of women prisoners. The silence about prison rape has been broken and we are learning what a widespread and horrible trauma it is for women prisoners. Human Rights Watch investigated the sexual abuse of women in five state prison systems from 1994 to 1996 and discovered widespread occurrences of rape and sexual harassment by male staff in all five. They did not compile any incidence figures, explaining that fears about retaliation and a lack of meaningful grievance procedures prevent a large number of rape survivors from reporting ongoing abuse by staff.

The survivor of prison rape is in a bind. Should he report the incident and risk the retaliation against "snitches" that the prison code mandates? Should she report the staff member and risk further abuse from him or his friends? The prisoner is confronted with complicated questions involving his safety and survival at precisely the moment when, just after experiencing a massive trauma, he is totally incapable of processing the event and rationally planning his next move. The aftereffects of prison rape include posttraumatic stress disorder, an inability to participate effectively in work assignments, drug counseling, and classes while inside, and a very high likelihood of social failure and re-arrest after release.

## Rape in Men's Prisons

Prison rape is about domination. One is either a "real man" who subdues and rapes an adversary, or one is a "punk." For the rape victim, reporting the assault to security staff is not a simple matter. The staff will demand that the victim identify the perpetrator before they will do anything. But the code requires that a prisoner must remain silent. If an inmate who has been raped cooperates with security staff in apprehending the man who raped him, the perpetrator might retaliate by killing the "snitch" or by arranging for another inmate to kill him even if the victim asks to "lock up" or voluntarily transfer to protective custody.

Prisoners have to be willing to fight to protect their honor, or they risk appearing weak and being raped. One way to avoid a fight is to look like you are very willing to fight. So prisoners lift weights compulsively, adopt the meanest stare they can muster, and keep their fears and their pain carefully hidden beneath a well-rehearsed tough-guy posture. Another way to avoid a fight is to join a clique or a gang. Mentally ill prisoners find it very difficult to navigate in this treacherous terrain, especially if they are not very tough. And many of them lack the social skills to join with others for self-protection. This leaves them especially vulnerable to sexual assault.

## The Perpetrator

The potential victim is not the only one who is terrified upon arriving in prison. Terror on the part of the prison rapist can be as great. But the perpetrator reacts differently, by brutalizing others before he becomes a victim himself. Fear motivates the taunting and testing of new arrivals as they enter their assigned tier. Who is this new inmate? Is he a "top dog" or a "punk"? It is as though the more veteran prisoners are wondering whether the new guy will topple them from their position or provide another conquest to consolidate their status. Even a small and fair young "fish" could turn out to be a "crazy" and kill his attacker. For example:

> A muscular African-American man of average size from the general population at a high-security prison tells me that in the holding tank on the way to prison he got into a fight with another man, beat him up, banged his head on the concrete a few times, and then sodomized him. I ask why he had to commit rape after winning the fight. First he tells me, with a laugh, it was because he was horny. I look at him quizzically, and he adds that wasn't really it, "It's just that's what you gotta do—if you don't do it, you haven't really won the fight."
>
> This is the first time he's been sent up to do "hard time." All his previous sentences were in the youth authority or county jail, and he was just trying to do the right thing to establish himself in prison. And it was the first time he ever raped anyone, woman or man. He believed that if he did not fight and win, and sodomize his vanquished foe, he would be considered a weakling and be treated by others the way he had treated the inmate he raped. Only after a few more rounds of questioning did he admit some remorse for having beaten and humiliated his rival so brutally. He confessed he was very nervous about going to prison.

The posturing that is required by the prison code, and the violent act of sexually dominating another man, provide the perpetrator with some semblance of manliness. And just as youths on the street gain the respect of other youths by brutalizing and humiliating crime victims or raping women, prison toughs prove their manliness and gain the respect of their peers by raping and humiliating weaker convicts.

In a large majority of prison rapes the perpetrator is a prisoner. But cases are surfacing in which a male staff-member rapes a prisoner. For instance, in 1990, Maurice Mathie, a thirty-year-old gay man, was raped by Sgt. Roy Fries at the Suffolk County Correctional Facility in New York. The correctional officer, an older man, had befriended Mathie. But after the prisoner began to trust him and tell him his troubles, Sgt. Fries made sexual advances. When Mathie resisted, the officer wrestled him into submission, handcuffed him to the pipes in a cell, and sodomized him. Mathie, who has suffered from anxiety, nightmares, and flashbacks since the rape, was eventually awarded $750,000 in a civil lawsuit he launched against the New York Department of Corrections for their "deliberate indifference."

## The Victim

The male prisoner who is raped struggles with inner voices saying he is no longer a man, he has been turned into a woman. Prisoners say he has been "turned out." Typically, a tougher prisoner forces a new arrival to become his "woman," and announces to the other prisoners that this new inmate is henceforth known as a punk and shall be available as a sexual object.

There are three parts to this dark mini-drama: The rapist has proven his manliness and reaffirmed his status as nonpunk in the dominance hierarchy. The prisoner who has been "turned out" is forced to join the ranks of prison punks. And in the process a public spectacle has occurred, a ritual of sorts, wherein the legitimacy of the dominance hierarchy has been reasserted and celebrated, to the disgrace of the victim.

Prison provides a dark mirror, a parody really, of gender relations in society at large. Outside prison, men battle for dominance and abuse women. With no women available, the same sensibility, but intensified in the way that every form of meanness is exacerbated in overcrowded prisons, is played out in acts of male-on-male sexualized violence. But the inmate rape victim, the "punk," is no longer a man in the eyes of the toughs; he has been turned into a woman. He is at the very bottom of the heap, precisely where men in and out of prison are trying their best to keep from falling.

For men, the lifelong obsession with hierarchies and domination goes all the way back to that schoolyard fight scenario. There was the winner, perhaps a bully, and the loser —the ninety-eight-pound weakling, the sissy, the chicken. Before long, the guy at the bottom is called a faggot or a girl. In a particularly vicious version, the loser's pants are pulled down and his genitals are mocked. There is an implicit threat of violence, even rape. For a certain number of men, it's not all fantasy; we are only beginning to discover how many men were sexually abused as boys.

In prison, those who fall to the bottom of the heap are severely abused. The trick for someone who is not a tough guy is to find a "third alternative," neither king of the mountain nor bottom of the heap. For instance, some frail intellectuals make themselves invaluable to other inmates by becoming knowledgeable about law and learning their way around the law library. They become immune to gladiatorial battles because they have a commodity to sell—jailhouse lawyers are much in demand in correctional settings where the inmates would like to win *habeus corpus* appeals of their convictions—so the prison toughs leave them alone.

Many prisoners who are slight and fair find other ways to avoid rape, sometimes by becoming the voluntary partner of a tougher convict. Once, while touring a prison in the Midwest, I encountered a male prisoner dressed as a woman. He told me that he had decided to become a woman soon after entering prison because, as a frail, young, blond "fish" he was subject to sexual abuse on a daily basis, whereas when he dressed as a woman and agreed to be the sexual partner of a strong prisoner he was granted protection.

Later that day I met with a group of security officers and the subject of this prisoner's cross-dressing came up. One officer said that had he seen "the lad" when he entered the prison, he would have given him this bit of advice: "What you want to do is the first time you go out on the yard you break off a metal bed post and shove it down your trouser leg. Then, when a big guy comes up and pinches your ass or makes a lewd remark, you pull out the metal stick and smack him as hard as you can across the face. You'll both get thrown in the hole for ten days. Then, when you get out, everyone will respect you as a 'crazy' and no one will hassle you for sex any more."

The rape victim, or punk, is not only subject to repeated brutalizations and rapes, he is also likely to be made into some tougher inmate's "slave." A slave not only provides sexual gratification on demand in exchange for protection, he also has to do whatever his owner demands of him, whether washing clothes and cleaning toilets or having sex with other prisoners when his owner demands it. There is even an organized sex industry in many men's prisons, comparable to the sex industry on the outside except that the prostitutes are men. Of course, some women are treated as brutally on the outside, in marriages or long-term relationships with a batterer, but even they can run to a battered women's shelter—not easily, of course, but there is a route. In prison, there is nowhere to turn.

Is it any wonder so many men who have been raped eventually commit suicide or suffer psychiatric decompensations? The situation is desperate, and desperate situations breed desperate acts. For instance:

> James Dunn, a prisoner at Angola State Prison in Louisiana, was raped when he entered the facility and forced into becoming his rapist's slave. After several years his "old man" was released, and Dunn decided to stop being a punk. But once a punk, always a punk in the eyes of the other cons, so after his owner's release other prison toughs approached Dunn for sex. Every time a different pris-

oner tried to claim him as a sex slave, Dunn had to fight for his honor and his life.

Eventually, in order to put an end to the daily fights and repeated injuries, he killed one of the would-be slave-owners. This put an end to the assaults, but he was sentenced to thirteen months in solitary confinement and had six years added to his sentence for the murder. After getting out of the hole, Dunn turned his energy to helping new arrivals at the institution learn the ropes and avoid sexual assaults and enslavement.

## Shame and Isolation

Usually a man who has been raped tries his best to keep it secret. Shame plays a big part, not only in victims' refusal to report rapes, but also in maintaining their isolation. When a boy is shamed, for instance by an alcoholic father or critical mother, he goes to his room—he does not seek the support of other members of the family. On the schoolyard, the boy who loses a fight or "chickens out" does not seek the support of his friends to heal his wounds, he stays to himself and the wounds fester. Shame leads to isolation, and in isolation there is little hope of transcending shame.

Stephen (Donny) Donaldson was an exception to the rule about men being silenced by shame. The founder and president of the organization Stop Prisoner Rape, Donny died of AIDS-related illness on July 18, 1996. He was infected with AIDS as a result of being raped on multiple occasions in jail and prison. Donaldson has written with great candor and eloquence about the traumas he experienced behind bars. Instead of keeping quiet about the humiliating treatment he received at the hands of jail and prison staff as well as other prisoners, "Donny the Punk" publicized his experience in an effort to stop prisoner victimization. He wrote an amicus brief to the Supreme Court in *Farmer* v. *Brennan*, a 1994 case that established the duty of prison officials to protect felons from unnecessary risk of sexual assault. Donaldson was interviewed widely and was featured in a 1996 prison rape segment on CBS' *Sixty Minutes*.

It can be very dangerous to speak frankly to other prisoners about one's traumas and pains. Again, the code. After being defeated in a fight, especially if he is raped, a man usually stays to himself. Perhaps he remains in his cell all day in the dark. But this is exactly the response that deepens depression or leads to the chronicity of posttraumatic stress disorders.

## Rape in Women's Prisons

There are cases of same-sex rape in women's prisons in which the perpetrator is another prisoner or a female staff member, and there have been reports of male staff raping female staff. But the vast majority of rapes in women's prisons involve a male staff member and a woman prisoner. The following example, though shocking, is fairly typical:

> While incarcerated at Dwight Correctional Center in Illinois, Zelda was raped repeatedly by a correctional officer. The first time, he entered her cell at night, hit her in the face, handcuffed her to her bed, and raped her vaginally and anally. Then he took off the handcuffs and left her cell. She was taken to the emergency room of a local hospital where a physical exam revealed she had been raped. She was returned to her cell and raped twice more by the same guard. No real investigation ever occurred, and he was never punished.

Often women prisoners "consent" to sex with a staff member. But is it really consensual? As when a male prisoner "consents" only to avoid further beatings, women who consent to ongoing sexual liaisons with staff members are actually doing so under a certain amount of unstated coercion.

A prisoner in a California women's facility tells me that quite a few women prisoners have sex with guards and other staff:

> They feel so isolated in prison, so guilty, they try in any way they can to feel loved—some just want to get daddy's approval—so they give in to guys hitting on them, bringing them flowers or little trinkets. They do it in an empty cell or a storage closet. Then, when they get pregnant, all hell breaks loose. The guard gets fired, the woman is thrown in the hole until she gives them permission to do an abortion, and then the whole thing gets hushed up and she's left to feel ashamed and afraid to tell anyone about it. Then she gets depressed but can't get to see a shrink because those guys don't really do anything but give out pills.

Women who go to prison are very likely to have been physically or sexually abused as children and to have been the victims of assault, domestic violence, or rape as adults. This makes the abuse they receive in prison seem "all too familiar," a reenactment of past traumas. In many cases, a major factor in their drug use and criminal activities was the wish to escape from an abusive, impossible situation. Then they were sent to prisons where more than half of the staff are male. Many women who are raped in prison are so accustomed to sexual exploitation that they are not aware of their rights and are very uncertain about precisely what constitutes sexual harassment or rape.

When women become pregnant after engaging in sexual intercourse with male staff members, they are usually treated harshly. In many institutions, they are given a term in solitary as punishment for their actions—or they might be told confinement in solitary is "for your protection." However, even when there is a nursery inside the prison, for instance at Bedford, when a woman prisoner who has been impregnated by a correctional officer applies to keep her baby in the nursery, her request is denied and she is forced to give up the baby.

When the administration is interested in preventing further sexual liaisons between staff and inmates, they pressure the pregnant woman to identify the father. If she does not want to identify him out of fear of retaliation, they place her in punitive segregation. If the woman goes to the medical staff she will probably be coerced into having an abortion.

Even when the legal requirements are followed and the woman is told about the benefits and risks of the procedure and asked for her informed consent, there are subtle and not-so-subtle coercive influences. For instance, she might be called into the warden's office and told how stupid it would be for her to carry the baby to term, or guards and counselors might harass her with daily lectures about her irresponsibility.

## Staff Collusion

The high incidence of rape in prison isn't due entirely to the cruelty of the perpetrators. The way the prison is run has much to do with the incidence of rape. If the warden is insensitive to prisoners' needs and the staff are never punished for acting sadistically toward prisoners, a certain tolerance for rape and sexual harassment evolves. If the warden and staff adopt an attitude of zero tolerance, however, and crack down forcefully on known perpetrators, the perpetrators have to stop exhibiting their dominance in such sadistic ways.

I have heard from quite a few male prisoners that they've reported to correctional officers that they were raped only to have the officer insist that they report the name of the assailant. One young man, a slender, passive fellow who was clearly suffering from acute schizophrenia with active hallucinations and delusions of persecution when I found him in a prison administrative segregation unit, told me that he had been raped by a member of a prison gang. He said that he had been confused at the time of the rape. I asked if he meant that he was suffering some of the same symptoms that were in evidence on the day of our interview. He nodded his head affirmatively and added that he was hearing voices at the time of the rape. Having newly arrived in the prison, and being terrified, he asked a correctional officer what he should do. The correctional officer told him he could not help unless he named the inmate who raped him.

The man cried at this point in his story and said he had made a big mistake. He snitched and now the gang wanted to kill him. The correctional officers moved him to administrative segregation because, though he was acutely psychotic, the prison psychiatric assessment team had decided his psychosis was not serious enough to warrant admission to the psychiatric hospital within the prison walls. Even though this man was in a single cell, he was on the same tier as members of the very gang whose member had raped him. The man was clinically paranoid; he was also in grave danger.

In regard to women's prisons, the collusion occurs when other staff members and administrators try to cover up the rape, or harass women who complain about being raped. But there are even instances in which the prior collusion of staff is what makes the rape possible.

For example, it recently came to light that a few male guards at the coeducational federal prison in Dublin, California, were accepting payment from male prisoners to leave the doors of women's cells unlocked so that male prisoners could enter and rape the women. The women sued the federal prison system, and the lawsuit was settled in early 1998. According to one of the women, "One [man] came into my room and tried to have sex with me. I kept telling him no and he just pulled my blouse down . . . and jumped on top of me." She further reports that when federal investigators interviewed her about the incident, "They said this is nothing new and we should just let it die down."

## Rape and Posttraumatic Stress Disorder

The first step in treating a traumatized rape victim is to help her establish a sense of safety. The survivor of rape has to be assured she is not subject to further attack by the perpetrator. Only when the survivor of a severe trauma feels safe to do so—and this means she has a sufficient support network and feels that her boundaries are fully intact and respected—is it useful to begin processing memories of the traumatic event. In this light, there is the potential for immense harm when prison staff insist that the victim of rape identify the perpetrator, or when the male guard who raped a woman prisoner continues to wield total control over every aspect of her life in prison. The subsequent posttraumatic stress disorder can be quite debilitating and long-lasting.

## Treatment for PTSD

Symptoms of PTSD follow a severe trauma that overwhelms the individual's capacity to feel in control of his life, to feel connected with others, and to be able to make sense of it all. As I mention in Chapter Two, the symptoms fall into two groups: intrusive and constrictive. *Intrusive symptoms* include flashbacks, nightmares, hyperarousal, startle, hypervigilance, and panic. The raw, unintegrated memories keep intruding, as though attacking from outside.

*Constrictive symptoms* include emotional numbing, social isolation, a curtailing of activities, and limitation on the places one is willing to venture. The victim of trauma is first overwhelmed by intrusive images related to the trauma; then she attempts to modulate the intensity of the experience by shutting down, initiating the constrictive symptomatology. But images and feelings related to the trauma soon break through in the form of flashbacks and nightmares, in spite of the attempt to numb and constrict. Then there are further attempts to shut down and modulate the intensity of the experience.

Most people experience oscillations between intrusive and constrictive symptoms in the wake of severe trauma. Ideally, over time, the oscillations diminish in severity, mourning and healing take place, the traumatic event is integrated into the individual's psychological meaning system, and the individual returns to the kinds of feelings, relationships, activities, and freedom to move about that characterized daily life prior to the trauma.

Some people are unable to mourn fully or integrate the traumatic event. For them, the oscillations continue unabated. At one moment they are subject to flashbacks, nightmares, panic attacks, or intense startle reactions. At another moment they are "closed down," afraid to go anywhere, see anyone, or do anything. They are suffering from PTSD. Sometimes individuals suffering from PTSD are so successful at numbing the intrusive symptoms that constrictive symptoms predominate. Of course, if the traumatic trigger to the clinical picture is not recognized, these individuals are assigned a diagnosis of depression.

If significant symptoms and incapacities last longer than a year after the trauma, PTSD is considered chronic. The progression of PTSD into a chronic phase is caused largely by a lack of opportunity to talk through the trauma in a supportive environment. Perhaps the traumatized individual was never able to establish sufficient safety and control of her boundaries to proceed with the working through, or perhaps an incapacity to talk about inner, psychological life prevented the person from telling the story. In any case, isolation following a severe trauma is to be avoided. The traumatic memories merely fester, thus leading to chronicity.

The oscillation between intrusive and constrictive states permits a certain amount of natural recovery through mourning and psychological integration. But if that natural process is punctuated by repeats of the same or similar kinds of trauma—beatings in the case of domestic violence, continuing sexual harassment and rapes in the case of prisoners—there is no opportunity for natural healing to occur. Instead, the repeated traumas intensify the intrusive symptoms as well as the need to constrict.

In addition, captivity brings the victim into prolonged contact with the perpetrator, whether he is a battering husband, a child's abuser, or the prison guard who repeatedly rapes a prisoner. In all of these cases, the feeling of safety is never consolidated, the remembering and working through are never possible, and the victim becomes permanently scarred by the repetitive traumas.

## A Case of PTSD Following Rape

I was asked to give an expert opinion about a young man who was raped by two gang members in a protective custody unit of a county jail. He was suing the county for not providing adequate protection. I examined the man and reviewed his file, including school reports and past psychiatric records. There seemed to be a pattern of vulnerability. For instance, as a mean prank, classmates had on occasion "suckered" him into doing things at school that would lead to punishment, and then laughed at him for being stupid enough to get caught.

In fact, he was in jail awaiting trial for a robbery that a couple of more savvy youths had talked him into committing with them. He was the only one who was caught, but he gave the police the names of his accomplices at the time of his arrest. He asked to be placed in protective custody because he feared he would be killed if other prisoners found out he had "snitched." This hapless young man was clearly a potential victim.

I examined him months after the incident and after he had been released from jail. He complained of daily flashbacks to the prison rape scene, nightmares, insomnia, fear of leaving his house, panic whenever he encountered strange men, and severe depression. After examining him I concluded that he was suffering from severe post-traumatic stress disorder, the causative trauma being the jail rape.

How was it possible in a protective custody unit for two gang members who had spent many years in prison to rape a vulnerable man who had never been to prison and never committed a violent crime? The two men who raped him were much bigger and stronger than he was, and had been returned from state prison to this jail only because they had to go to court to stand trial for gang-related violence inside prison. But they'd been "outed" by their gangs. In other words, they were in trouble with their gangs, perhaps because they were perceived as snitches, and since they were in grave danger anywhere in the correctional system they were placed in protective custody.

At the time of the rape, a single officer was on duty in the large protective custody unit. She was responsible for "observing" a dayroom, a dining area, and two floors of cells with open doors. It was not possible at any given time for that officer to observe the entire unit, and in fact the victim told me that the rape took place over a forty-five minute time span in a second-floor cell while the officer was sitting at a desk in the dayroom and unable to see inside the cells above her head. The two perpetrators lured the young man into a second-floor cell by offering to share their pruno (jail brew) with him. After several drinks, the two larger men told the victim to take his pants off, they wanted to have some fun. When he refused and tried to get up to leave the cell, they hit him several times in the face and forced him to lie face-down on the bunk. They proceeded to rip his pants off and each took several turns raping him while the other held him down and pressed his mouth into a pillow to keep him quiet.

Of course, the victim shouldn't have been housed with the men who raped him. But in an overcrowded system it's unlikely that inmates of different security levels will be further segregated once it is decided they need protective custody—the staff are so far behind classifying the new inmates that the assignment to protective custody is considered classification enough. In this case, either the jail facility needs to create security levels within the protective custody units so that hard-core gang members cannot be thrown together with inmates who are unable to defend themselves, or the staff needs to supervise the inmates more closely. That would require more staff.

## Replaying the Trauma

Advocates for women who have been raped complain that the victims are subjected to even worse trauma at the hands of insensitive police officers, harried emergency room doctors, and attorneys who grill them about their past sexual experiences in the courtroom. Essentially, the trauma of rape is replayed in the course of insensitive postrape treatment.

There is another issue involved in the replay of trauma. Continuing with the analogy of rape in the community, a woman rape victim who was sexually molested as a girl tends to suffer worse psychiatric symptoms following the rape than does a woman who had not suffered prior sexual abuse. Similarly, if the inmate who is raped by another inmate has a history of brutalization and rape at the hands of a violent, alcoholic stepfather, then he will probably not tolerate the new trauma very well at all.

We know that prisoners, on average, suffered a great amount of abuse prior to incarceration. And obviously prison life is rife with new traumas, many even more severe than the ones the average prisoner suffered earlier. The prisoner probably experiences rape as a replay of the abuse he suffered early on. When correctional staff treat the victims of rape or other varieties of prison trauma in an insensitive or brutal manner, the psychic damage is compounded.

## HIV and AIDS

The incidence of AIDS in prison in 1994 was 518 cases per 100,000, compared to a comparable annual incidence in the total population of 31 cases per 100,000. This fifteen-fold greater incidence is not surprising, considering how much crime is drug-related, and how prevalent AIDS is among intravenous drug users. In prison, HIV is transmitted by drug use, tattooing, and sex. Most states refuse to provide condoms to prisoners, as though supplying condoms would signal support for sexual activities. And educational programs, which have proved very effective at decreasing high-risk sexual behaviors on the outside, are not a priority in most departments of corrections.

HIV testing and isolation of prisoners who test positive is a complicated matter in prison. For instance, there was a policy in California prisons in the late 1980s whereby a prison physician could test a prisoner for HIV without obtaining his informed consent, and all prisoners found to be HIV-positive were transferred automatically to a segregated AIDS cellblock, whether or not they exhibited symptoms or qualified for a diagnosis of AIDS. The prisoner had to leave the prison or cellblock where he'd been housed. He probably lost his prison job. His HIV status became known to the entire prison population. Once in the AIDS unit, he would no longer be permitted on the large prison yard but had to make use of a much smaller and ill-equipped yard attached to the AIDS unit. In addition, he was likely to be double-celled with a prisoner who was suffering from AIDS, and he was surrounded by emaciated prisoners dying of AIDS-related illnesses.

In 1989, while testifying in *Gates* v. *Deukmejian*, I was asked about the psychiatric effects of that policy. I explained there were problems with the policy at each step of the process. Informed consent is an important issue in identifying people who are HIV-positive. When blood tests are conducted without the prisoner's consent, he is likely to feel abused and disrespected. When a person hears he is HIV-positive, he needs time to digest the news and figure out how it will affect his life. But if he is immediately thrown into a cellblock with prisoners who are already sick and dying, he is deprived of the opportunity to decide whom he wants to tell about his status and which of his ongoing activities he wants to alter or curtail. The terror evoked by the diagnosis is exacerbated by his gruesome situation and restricted activities. Whether he is prone to panic attacks or depression, his emotional distress is intensified and some form of emotional breakdown is very likely. Not surprisingly, there were several suicides reported in that AIDS cellblock.

The federal judge in *Gates* v. *Deukmejian* ordered an end to the involuntary blood tests and required the California Department of Corrections to give asymptomatic prisoners who tested positive the choice of whether to go to the designated cellblock. He also ordered that HIV-positive prisoners be permitted access to all appropriate work and recreational programs, and be provided adequate medical and psychiatric care. Policies vary from state to state, but some states still perform mandatory HIV testing without prisoners' informed consent, and some states isolate prisoners who test positive.

In this light, consider the plight of the prisoner who is raped, converts to HIV-positive, and is sent to a crowded, dark cellblock where activities are greatly restricted. The harsh treatment constitutes a retraumatization that is likely to magnify the damage done by the sexual assault and to impair the prisoner's capacity to work through the experience of rape and return to full emotional functioning. In any case, the risk of HIV infection greatly magnifies the damage done by rape and exaggerates the terror connected with sexual assault.

## Postrelease Adjustment

Many prisoners' lives have been destroyed by prison rape. We never even hear about the less dramatic survivors who, whatever the degree of postrelease success they attain, suffer ever after from terrifying flashbacks and a deep-seated incapacity to trust others. It is inspiring to hear occasionally of a survivor, such as Donny Donaldson, who goes on to defy the commandment to suffer in silence. Donaldson has had an impact. The organization he founded, Stop Prisoner Rape, continues to draw public attention to the hellish inferno our prisons have become. The Human Rights Watch investigation into sexual abuse of women prisoners has also helped.

Unfortunately, many male victims of rape become perpetrators as soon as they get the opportunity. I witnessed an example of this "identification with the oppressor" while serving in the capacity of consultant to a community halfway house for individuals with chronic and severe mental disorders. The staff was very concerned about a series of incidents involving a twenty-five-year-old African-American man of average size. He was discovered pressuring vulnerable female residents into having sex with him, while he repeatedly confronted male residents as well as strangers on the street, demanding they stop staring at him unless they wanted to fight. Obviously his aggressive behavior was making life difficult for the women, as well as dangerous for him and the other men.

I asked the staff whether this young man had served any time behind bars, and it turned out he had spent quite a bit of time in jail and prison. I suggested that his counselor might enquire tactfully whether he had ever been raped. It turned out that he had, repeatedly. He was too ashamed to talk about it, but clearly he was compensating for having been a victim by victimizing others, all the while obsessing about his manliness. One wonders how many dangerous predators our correctional system is producing.

Women who have been raped and brutalized are much less likely to take their hostility out on someone else. Instead, they turn it inward and become depressed. Women survivors of prison rape also tend to suffer from unexpressed rage, low self-esteem, various forms of anxiety, and a wide variety of emotional symptoms.

For both male and female survivors, the postrape psychiatric symptoms continue long after they are released, and cause severe disability. I have seen quite a few survivors of prison rape who returned to drugs, crime, or prostitution after they were released; and in every case they link their failures in life to the trauma of prison rape. Others find they cannot get out of their depression or their panic attacks long enough to take very good care of their offspring.

This ongoing social tragedy deserves much more public attention. We know that rape ruins victims' chances of reforming themselves inside and succeeding after they are released. We know what kind of mental health treatment is effective in preventing PTSD and minimizing the long-term disability caused by sexual assault. We are also aware of the kinds of staff collusion that permit repeated rapes to occur, and we know what prison administrators can do to reduce the incidence of prison rape as well as the long-term emotional damage. There is no excuse for continued collusion and inaction.

---

Quality visitation, the subject of the next chapter, seems to reduce the prevalence of rape behind bars and to improve the mental health of prisoners. Men and women prisoners who remain in close touch with their families are less prone to be involved in sexual assaults and are less vulnerable to psychiatric decompensation.

# 7

# Lack of Contact with Loved Ones

Regular visits from loved ones help prisoners do their time, maintain emotional stability, avoid disciplinary infractions, and adjust in the community after release. In the absence of quality visitation, prisoners are more prone to mental distress. Prisoners who suffer from serious and persistent mental illnesses deteriorate further from the lack of loving contact. In this sense, correctional policies that decrease the number and quality of visits worsen the mental health crisis behind bars.

Compare a prisoner who is cut off entirely from family and friends and another who enjoys weekly visits with his wife and children. It is not difficult to predict which prisoner, all other factors being equal, is more likely to stay out of trouble while locked up and which is more likely to suffer emotional breakdowns, run into disciplinary problems in the pen, and then fall back into a life of family instability, drugs, and crime when he returns to the community. Research shows that continuous contact with family members throughout a prison term makes it much less likely that a prisoner will be re-arrested and reimprisoned in the years following his release. Prisoners tend to be more content, and more capable of maintaining their sanity, if they stay in close contact with loved ones outside.

Unfortunately, there seems to be a wish among a lot of respectable citizens to "disappear" convicts. They rest easier once offenders have been "sent up," and they don't want to hear anything further about the men and women who are locked behind bars. Out of sight, out of mind. With little or no public concern about keeping prisoners in contact with their families, departments of correction are free to institute new policies that make visits ever more difficult. Little thought is given to the hardships this creates for prisoners, their families, and their communities.

## The Benefits of Quality Visitation

The quality of visitation during a convict's term correlates strongly with his capacity to participate in the program inside the walls and to make a successful adjustment in the community after his term ends. Conversely, a lack of quality visitation makes it much more likely the prisoner will get into disciplinary trouble or suffer from mental illness.

### Some Benefits

Research involving visitation and recidivism demonstrates an obvious correlation. For instance, in one study, 50 percent of prisoners who did not receive visits from family members were re-arrested in the year following release and 12 percent were reimprisoned, but 70 percent of prisoners who were visited regularly by at least three people while serving their term were free of arrests during their first postrelease year, and only 2 percent were reimprisoned.

Quality visits reduce the likelihood that a prisoner will get into a violent altercation. For instance, a twenty-eight-year-old male prisoner confides that when his wife fails to visit him for several weeks, or when he is unable to reach her by phone, he becomes jealous and thinks she might have found another man: "Then I get mean, you know what I mean? I carry a chip on my shoulder, and the first guy to say the wrong thing, I'm just raring to turn and slug him. If it happens to be a guard, I'm in big trouble—I get thrown in the hole, lose my job, and they add a lot of time to my sentence."

Another man tells me it was only after they moved him from a prison near his home to one on the other side of the state, and his sweetheart told him she would no longer be able to visit as often, that he began experiencing bouts of extreme jealousy and had great difficulty controlling his rage. Other prisoners report that they are extremely stressed by the fact they are unable to maintain close contact with their children. A thirty-year-old African-American man confides that his father was in prison while he was "comin' up," and several of the men his mother lived with during those years beat him, one even raped his sister. So now, while he is locked up and unable to protect his son (eight years) and daughter (seven), and his wife is threatening to leave him for a man who can provide for her and the kids, he feels a huge amount of shame for having left his children unprotected in the same way his father left him.

There is debate about the utility and safety of conjugal visits. Conjugal visits occur in a designated area of the prison where the prisoner and his loved ones are left alone in a somewhat private, apartment-like setting, for several hours or overnight. There may be a kitchen in the unit. There may be several bedrooms for prisoners' families with children. Forty percent of family visits involve family members other than a romantic partner.

Critics say this kind of visitation constitutes "coddling." Some correctional personnel say it creates security problems or requires too much staff time. Advocates of such visits counter that there are many benefits in keeping inmates connected with loved ones, including the fact that prisoners must earn the privilege of conjugal visits and this makes them more willing to cooperate with the institution's rules and programs. A study of California's Family Visiting Program found that 90 percent of staff members endorsed the program. Of course, the maintenance of a quality conjugal visiting program requires certain resources. But the benefits far outweigh the costs.

Consider the issue of prison rape in men's prisons. Conjugal visits are not frequent or regular enough to significantly decrease male prisoners' sexual appetites. But prison staff tell me that a man who is permitted even intermittent conjugal visits with his wife or sweetheart is less likely to engage in violent sex with other men. Perhaps periodic conjugal visits help a man continue to believe he is lovable, or perhaps they serve to bolster his sense of manliness.

Connection with loved ones also helps prisoners keep an eye on getting out, and this may explain why they do not feel as much need to get into fights or participate in dangerous sex. Perhaps the most important gain is continued intimacy. Women prisoners tend to make kids a higher priority anyway, but for men as well as women, regular visitation with families is crucial not only for them, but for the next generation as well. It is unwise on many counts to rip prisoners from their families and friends. Close contact with family and loved ones definitely mitigates against meanness, madness, and despair.

## Contact via Correspondence

As one of three co-editors of a book on men in prison, *Confronting Prison Masculinities: The Gendered Politics of Punishment* (Temple University Press, 1999), I have been corresponding with prisoner/writers around the country. In response to ads that we placed in periodicals, prisoners submit manuscripts for consideration. We review their writings and correspond with them. In quite a few cases, even if a prisoner's writing is not appropriate for the book, the man writes back that what he really needs is a friend. Usually there is an urgency in his plea.

One male prisoner wrote that it is impossible to sustain friendships inside prison. All his old friends have either died, gone to prison themselves, or forgotten about him. The plea for friendship is usually accompanied by inflated praise: "Terry, you're the only person in the whole world who I can trust." Another man writes: "I feel you, I know you're the kind of person who would never betray a friend." I feel a combination of sadness and fear as I read letters like these: sadness about the misery and loneliness the prisoner reports, fear about a friendship that is so young and tentative and yet already so important to him. Will the passion and exaggeration turn to rage if I disappoint him?

Once, after I had been corresponding with an inmate for several months, commenting on his poetry and sending him stamps, one of my letters was delayed in the prison mailroom. The next thing I knew I received an angry letter from him saying it's OK if I don't want to write to him anymore, but I should send back all of his poetry. We straightened out the miscommunication and decided that the mailroom delay was probably due to inefficiency and not, in this case at least, to any kind of plot on the part of the correctional authorities to sabotage our correspondence. But the intensity of the disappointment and brittleness of this and other such relationships cause me to consider carefully the pros and cons of commencing any ongoing correspondence with a prisoner. And when I do begin to write consistently, I try my best to keep expectations realistic and then to avoid disappointing my correspondent.

When such things are taken into consideration, corresponding with prisoners can be very rewarding. I recommend it. In fact, if more people on the outside corresponded with prisoners, the prisoners would feel less isolated, perhaps they might even try harder to overcome the odds against successful integration into the community after they are released.

## Visitation and Mental Illness

Repeatedly I discover in the histories of prisoners who become psychotic or commit suicide that some form of heightened separation from loved ones precipitated the breakdown. Sometimes it's a wife who deserts the imprisoned husband, but often it is simply the failure of family members to make the longer trek to visit the inmate following his transfer to a facility further from home.

As I mention in Chapter Five, many women prisoners fall into a deep depression when they are moved to a prison that makes visitation with their children problematic. For instance, a thirty-two-year-old Mexican-American woman serving time for a drug offense in a federal prison explains: "When you see your kids each week at visiting times you know if they're being taken care of right—you can tell if they're being fed right or beaten or ignored—but when it's not possible to see them regularly, you start to worry more, the worries turn into nightmares, and you just feel lousy as a mother and afraid for your kids."

Mental health professionals are very aware of the importance of contact with loved ones. People who do not enjoy close intimacies present a greater risk for psychotic decompensation or suicide than those who do, inside or outside of prison walls. In the community, when a patient begins to decompensate or feel suicidal, it can be very helpful to contact family members, find out about stressful family dynamics, and, if possible, alleviate some of the current stress coming from the family. This might be accomplished with a couple therapy or family therapy session, or merely by the therapist making contact with an estranged family member to find out more about the patient and the reason for the estrangement.

In prison, there is far too little contact between mental health staff and prisoners' families. There are exceptions, of course. For instance, in prisons with model inpatient units, there is usually a social worker on the ward who makes an effort to contact the family to find out what news from home might have caused a prisoner's breakdown, and possibly to ask family members to come to the institution for family therapy. But in most cases, the mental health staff are too overwhelmed by their caseload to spend much time contacting family members. Most of the clinical charts I read in prisons make no mention of current family relationships. Many do not even contain a family history.

## Problems with the Visitation Policies

Of course, if a family member or loved one is imprisoned, there are discontinuities in family life and resulting hardships. This is meant to be a part of the punishment. Felons are separated from society, and that includes their families. But there are obstacles to quality visitation that go far beyond what is inherent in imprisonment itself. I have mentioned the tendency to situate correctional facilities far from prisoners' homes. There are other ways in which prison systems can and do make visiting more difficult than it needs to be.

## Harassing Visitors

Visitors to prisons are routinely searched and made to stand in lines prior to their visit. A certain amount of searching is required for security reasons. But sometimes staff make it excessively difficult for visitors, for instance by subjecting them to crude insults as they go through the gates or by making them go through a strip search and orifice examination prior to their visit. And the wait can be long, typically an hour or two.

There are other barriers. Prison mail is carefully scrutinized and censored—sometimes excessively and illegally. Prisoners are denied visits if they are being disciplined. Visitors are turned away if the staff feel their attire is not appropriate. Or they are turned away because there are too many visitors that day and visiting hours end before they get to the front of the line. A wife or mother might drive four hundred miles to see a prisoner only to be told she cannot visit that day or even the next. She is forced to return home without being able to see her loved one. There is a tendency for these visitors to leave the parking lot angry, perhaps swearing to themselves they will not be so quick to make the long trip again very soon. In these and many other ways, prisoners are cut off from their families and from society, and this makes their stay behind bars more difficult.

Moving prisoners from one institution to another, something that happens more often in overcrowded facilities, makes it difficult for the average prisoner to form lasting bonds with other prisoners and to stay in contact with loved ones on the outside. There is even a homeless population in some prison systems. Certain prisoners are moved from prison to prison so often that they spend more time on buses or sleeping in local county jails during transport than they spend in a prison cell. Ex-prisoner Dan Martin calls it "bus therapy." For these prisoners to get involved in any meaningful activity is impossible. Many go mad. It is rumored that guards use this kind of "bus therapy" as an informal (and thus nonappealable) punishment for convicts who disrespect or anger them. Since a prisoner who is en route cannot receive mail or phone calls, she can be held incommunicado for weeks or months while being shuffled from one prison to another.

In the early 1980s, the California Department of Corrections made the prospect of visiting a prisoner even more frightening by conducting mandatory searches of visitors' cars as they entered the prison parking lot. In preparation for testimony in a lawsuit filed by the prisoners' families, I interviewed several women whose cars were searched at the San Quentin prison parking lot during that period. They told me that once a vehicle entered the parking lot gate, its occupants were detained and searched, even if they did not consent and chose to leave without a visit. There was a small sign at the entrance to the visitors' parking lot stating that those who entered were subject to a search, which most people arriving at the lot failed to notice. Thus, even visitors who did not know they might be subjected to a search would not be permitted to turn around and leave in order to avoid the procedure.

The occupants of cars were forced to exit their car and undergo a body search as well as an examination of their purses and possessions. Dogs trained to smell drugs were then led through the vehicle while guards searched under seats, in glove compartments, and in trunks. Many visitors' cars were left a mess. If anything was turned up, the visitors would be arrested for violating state laws regarding prison visitation and would be denied visits to their family member for a long time.

In one case, a rusty, crumpled beer can was found in the trunk of an old car and the prisoners' wife and child were denied access to the prisoner for a year. In another case, a middle-aged mother of a prisoner was arrested for possession of narcotics and attempting to smuggle narcotics into a prison after the dogs sniffed a small roach (the butt of a marijuana cigarette) in the car's glove compartment. The mother's youngest son had left the roach there when he last borrowed the car.

The practice of searching visitors' cars and trucks in the parking lot did nothing to deter the drug supply inside the walls. Would a visitor really bring a rusty beer can or a roach from the glove compartment into the prison? But the average rate of visitation in the affected prisons showed a sharp decline while the searches were occurring. Attorneys for the prisoners as a class were able to demonstrate that the searches were not necessary for security reasons but constituted a cruel and unusual deprivation for the prisoners, and a settlement was reached that included discontinuation of the car searches.

California and several other states have recently begun to require visitors to undergo X-ray searches before entering the visiting area of certain prisons. Once again, whether this kind of search has any effect on the smuggling of contraband is questionable, but it certainly has the effect of cutting down on visitation. For instance, many potential visitors are concerned about the health effects of exposure to radiation.

## Visiting in Maximum Security

Visitation for prisoners in disciplinary segregation tends to be even more problematic. This is a very unfortunate development, since this is a group who actually need quality visits more than most if they are to rein in their hostility and do their time peacefully and constructively. But each step of an individual inmate's progress toward long-term housing in solitary confinement involves an incremental diminution in the quality and regularity of his contact with loved ones.

The more disciplinary infractions a prisoner acquires, the higher level security he is assigned, and often this means a transfer to a prison further from the prisoner's home community. Prisoners who hail from urban Detroit and receive a certain number of disciplinary tickets in any prison are sent to the maximum security prison at Marquette, about as far as one can travel from Detroit and still remain in Michigan. Prisoners from Philadelphia are sent to the State Correctional Institution at Greene, a drive of about six hours away. Similarly, California's highest security prison, Pelican Bay State Prison, is located in the northwest corner of the state, very far from San Diego and Los Angeles, cities called home by the majority of inmates at Pelican Bay. An African-American prisoner from South Central Los Angeles explained to me that he would like to see his "homeys," and they used to visit when he was awaiting trial in a local jail and even when he was imprisoned at Chino in Southern California, but since he has been transferred to Pelican Bay State Prison no one but his mother has the commitment to come and visit him, and even she cannot make the trip very often.

Once a prisoner is locked up in a segregated security unit, she loses the privilege of "contact visits." Prisoners locked in most security units can only see visitors through a thick pane of glass and have to talk over a phone. And there are other security precautions, including more stringent searches of visitors and more handcuffing and shackling of prisoners as they are led to and from visiting areas.

The prisoners stop envisioning a future in their family, so they don't write as often. Their wives and children are hurt, and make less contact. Then the prisoner becomes depressed, or rageful. And he is less able to do his program, more likely to get into a fight. The result is an unfortunate paradox: Prisoners who are deemed to have discipline problems are sent further from home, where they receive fewer and lesser quality visits; but with diminished quality contact with loved ones they are likely to grow even more desperate and rageful and get into even worse fights. The prisoners who have the hardest time controlling themselves are deprived of the very resource that might help them control themselves better.

If the aim of correctional policies is to attain peace and mental health in the prisons and help prisoners reform themselves and become law-abiding citizens, the tendency for visitation to be more problematic the higher the prisoner's security level is extremely counterproductive. Of course, requests for larger state corrections budgets to build more supermaximum prison units are always accompanied by dramatic reports of heightened violence between prisoners. It seems that corrections departments have a financial interest in causing the prisoners to fail—then they can justify more prison construction and higher operating budgets.

## A Prisoner and His Mother

A twenty-five-year-old white prisoner, K. R., and his mother testified in a federal class action suit against the California Department of Corrections. The litigation concerned the issues of overcrowding and other forms of "cruel and unusual punishment." K. R. and his mother were asked about the ordeal they suffered during his confinement at San Quentin. He had been convicted of robbery. There was no weapon, and no force was used. The victim handed over his wallet, which contained $38. For this first offense, he was sentenced to prison and spent a significant part of his term in administrative segregation. He did not have any disciplinary charges against him while in prison, so he was only placed in administrative segregation because of a series of boondoggles in the classification process. Asked what type of visits he was permitted while in solitary confinement, K. R. responded:

> ANSWER: Noncontact visits. You are put there in a little cell type area with a glass window and a telephone, and the visitor sits on the other side with the telephone.
>
> QUESTION: Were you shackled in any way?
>
> ANSWER: Yes, you was. You have waist chains on you, they take you from your block to the visiting, they put you in the little cell

area I'm talking about, and they release the shackles from you, the waist chains.

QUESTION: Would your visitors be able to see you in chains?

ANSWER: Yes, they could.

The attorney then asked him about his emotional state after he had been in solitary confinement with no exercise and only noncontact visits for eighteen days:

ANSWER: My emotional state, I was very humiliated, not being able to get out and exercise, my body was sore, but it is really humiliating, because you go to them visits and the people see you with chains and stuff on, it was like you are degraded, you know.

QUESTION: During the noncontact visits, were you able to communicate with your family?

ANSWER: Not really.

QUESTION: In what respects were you inhibited?

ANSWER: You couldn't really talk about getting out and getting help, because the phones are bugged and you don't know if you are going to say the wrong thing, if people are going to yank you out from the phone because you said something you are not supposed to. You don't know what to say, except "How are you doing? You are looking a lot better."

K. R. eventually suffered a nervous breakdown and became suicidal while in Administrative Segregation (Ad Seg) at San Quentin. After emergency psychiatric examination he was placed on suicide precautions for several days.

K. R.'s mother also testified in court. After describing the long waits in the visitors' line and the body searches that preceded visits, she was asked what the differences were between contact and noncontact visits. She responded from the witness stand: "The noncontact visits were very painful to go through because feeling and contacting of your loved one is an important part of giving them encouragement. There was a barrier there. We were not comfortable. We were told we couldn't say anything that we didn't want to be heard by everybody. And we spent a lot of time on the phones making light conversation that had nothing to do with immediate problems."

Later, K. R. was transferred to a low-security facility and had a contact visit with his mother and his five-year-old daughter. Up until the time of that visit, K. R. had instructed his mother to explain why his daughter could not visit him by lying to her and saying he was too sick. His mother described the first contact visit:

> And we waited for about a little over an hour, and I kind of kept her attention drawn and back turned and everything to anything that would resemble a prison type of thing. She lives on a military base, so officers and things were not of importance to her. And all of a sudden, I don't know why, I looked to the right, which was to the main visiting area, and I saw my son come walking through there. And I turned to Sarah, and I said, "There's your daddy." And she said, "He is not sick." And she went running over to him. And he didn't run to her, though. He stopped at the line, and she got over there. So we were thrilled to death. There was a lot of crying and emotional scenes and so on, but we were able to spend the visit in a regular area where he could hold her and talk to her.

QUESTION: Did having that contact visit have an effect on your son?

ANSWER: Yes, he was the best, probably, that he had been through this. It was highly important to him. And, of course, we could touch him, too. And our mouths were going, and we were telling everything we could think of and whispering and talking, and a tremendous relief that we didn't have to worry about what was happening, what was going—being overheard or anything like that.

K. R. spent only a month in solitary confinement. Think about the prisoners who are given an indeterminate term in "the hole." If K. R. developed an emotional disorder and became suicidal because of the stress, how much greater is the stress on someone who is "locked down" for a significantly longer period?

## Prisoners Who Refuse Visits

I have encountered quite a few prisoners in maximum and supermaximum security facilities who, like K. R., choose not to have their families visit. They discourage visits with their children because they do not want them to see their father in shackles. For example, I asked a black man serving a year in Indiana's supermaximum security prison at Westville whether his family comes to visit very often. "Never!" he says emphatically.

"Why not?" I ask. "Is it the distance they would have to travel?"

"Naw, they don't mind driving the hour it takes to get here, I just don't want them to see me like this."

I ask this man what he means and he explains that in every other prison where he has been the prisoners wear their own personal clothing and have contact visits, but in supermax they wear prison-issue jumpsuits and have to visit in a booth and talk on phones. He continues: "I have a hard enough time explaining to my kids why their daddy's in prison. I don't want them to remember me shackled and wearing a prison jumpsuit."

Many prisoners confined in lock-up units confide similar feelings. They miss their wives, their parents and their kids, but their pride makes them refuse visits. In Michigan, the questionnaire I sent to prisoners involved in *Cain* v. MDOC included the question: "Would the loss of your personal possessions and clothing change your ability to relate to family and friends?" The new policy at issue in that case would severely restrict prisoners' possessions and force them to wear uniforms. Here are a few typical responses from male prisoners:

> *I don't want my children and family to see me in a prison uniform.*
>
> *It will make you feel less when you visit.*
>
> *Shame, so yes.*
>
> *Yes, because they would not be needed. They like doing things for me, showing love.*
>
> *Yes. Because I've already been deprived of their companionship and now I can't have the stuff that keeps them in my thoughts.*
>
> *Yes, because it would open many doors to questions I would have to explain as to why I am upset, or why I wear the same clothes all the time.*

Here are a few representative responses from women prisoners:

> *Yes, I would not want them to see me that way.*
>
> *My family sent me items that helped them to walk this road with me. It is so hard to just try to tell a ninety-year-old mother she cannot send me just a small token of her love. I couldn't bear to see her without wearing the clothes she sent.*
>
> *Yes, they show love by sending me things I really need, and that would be lost.*
>
> *It is hard being in here and hard on our families. We have children that don't understand why we can't come home*

> *and to have to visit them in prison uniforms is even more confusing to them.*

A fifty-one-year-old mother of two and grandmother, serving three to fifteen years in a minimum security prison, writes:

> It is difficult enough for our family and children to see us in this situation. I am sure it would alter my desire to see my children and grandchildren. One of the things that we are encouraged to do is to reestablish family ties and to make improvements in our ability to communicate and conduct ourselves as responsible, productive people. Looking at the implementation of this policy in conjunction with so many others, it's as if it is becoming the department of correction's goal to simply throw away and forget those of us that happen to fall into their hands. Phone calls are no longer private, siblings are no longer allowed to bond, family are treated as if they are incarcerated when they visit loved ones. It is as if the primary goal of assisting an individual in the process of rebuilding their life has been overshadowed by the need to become totally punitive, and to contrive whatever means it takes to promote recidivism.

## Consequences for the Community

Prisoners are not the only ones who suffer from a lack of visitation. One tragic consequence of the imprisonment binge and the attempt to "disappear" the felon is the decimation of families. Whether the prisoners are men or women, their children get along much more poorly in their absence. We are witnessing a widespread intergenerational tragedy: A parent goes to prison and as a consequence a child falls into drugs, crime, and chronic failure, perhaps even prison some day.

It is never good for a community to have a large number of its young adults shipped off to prison. Consider the impact of the imprisonment binge on the inner-city, African-American community. There is talk of "family values" and the moral imperative for men to fulfill their promises to wives and children. But with over 30 percent of young African-American men under the jurisdiction of the criminal justice system, there are a large number of single mothers and single-parent households, and a short supply of men.

If the ex-prisoner returns to the community angrier, more emotionally distressed, and disconnected from family on account of the lack of quality visits, he is all the more likely to return to a life of drugs and crime—possibly more violent crimes than he committed prior to incarceration.

---

Barriers to quality visitation have a very harmful effect on prisoners' mental health. The lack of quality contact definitely worsens depressions. Prisoners who, because of mental illness, are prone to act out by breaking rules and becoming violent lose the moderating influence that close contact with family members could provide. Not accidentally, a significant number of prison suicides are precipitated by the discontinuation of contact with loved ones—a subject I take up in the next chapter.

# 8

# Prison Suicide

The suicide rate in prison is twice as high as in the general population, and the suicide rate in jail is approximately nine times as high as in the general population, or five times as high as in prison. This is a rough estimate, since the rate varies widely from state to state. Still, these figures give some indication that suicide is a major health hazard within correctional facilities.

Sadly, I have many personal stories of prisoner suicides to report. Each time I am asked to give an opinion about the quality of mental health services in a jail or prison, I request the charts of all recent suicides—the attempts as well as the ones that resulted in death. Then I interview the prisoners I am able to locate who have tried unsuccessfully to kill themselves. In cases of successful suicide, medical facilities usually carry out a "psychological autopsy," a postmortem clinical investigation of the case, and I ask to see the reports of these investigations for the past two or three years. The suicide attempts and deaths behind bars provide a portrait of despair among prisoners and a devastating critique of unfortunate staff attitudes and deficiencies in suicide prevention programs.

## A Tragic Epidemic

Though suicide is a big problem in jails and prisons, the patterns typical of the two kinds of correctional settings are different. Still another pattern is the invisible suicide that is labeled something else, for instance a deadly fight or a fatal escape attempt. Understanding the patterns and the reasons prisoners become desperate enough to take their own lives can help staff maintain the kind of vigilance that is needed if suicides are to be prevented.

## Suicide in Jail

In the late 1970s, partially in response to class action lawsuits charging inadequate mental health care in several U.S. jails, a spate of publications bemoaned the alarmingly high rate of suicide among prisoners. An amazing finding was that at least half of jail suicides occur within the first twenty-four hours after arrest, and a significant proportion within the first few hours. There is some evidence that pretrial jail detainees are more prone than sentenced prisoners to self-injury. The jail detainee has to cope with the shock of being arrested and deprived of freedom, the shame of it, and the frightening prospect of spending time behind bars.

The American Medical Association, the U.S. Department of Justice, and many states have issued standards for medical and mental health services in local detention facilities, including clear guidelines about the kinds of screening of incoming detainees and staff training that are required to detect prisoners at risk for suicide. For instance, since a large proportion of jail suicides occur in isolation cells, isolation is obviously not an effective way to manage potentially suicidal inmates and should be prohibited. Instead, direct observation is recommended, or at least rigorous every-fifteen-minute checks.

Today it is standard practice in most jails to screen incoming detainees for signs of suicide risk and for the non–mental health staff to undergo training in the recognition of prisoners who are at risk. Still, the incidence of jail suicide remains high. One of the reasons is that many counties adopt acceptable written protocols for screening and prevention but fail miserably when it comes to putting their protocols into practice.

## Suicide in Prison

Suicide accounts for more than half of the number of inmates dying in custody. In 1993, there were 26.4 suicides per 100,000 inmates in California's state prisons and 25 suicides per 100,000 inmates in the Texas system. The prison suicide rate in these two states, the states with the largest total prison populations, was approximately twice the rate for the general population that year. In the same year, the suicide rate in Georgia's prisons was 10.8 per 100,000, and in Florida it was 9.9—somewhat below the rate for the general population.

Unlike the pretrial jail detainee, the prison inmate has had time to adjust somewhat to the fate that awaits him, and worries more about being separated from loved ones and his ability to cope with a lengthy sentence in a brutal, hierarchical prison environment.

I have spoken to dozens of prisoners who have made serious suicide attempts and survived, and they have reported a variety of reasons for their self-destructive actions. One man told me that his release date was getting close, and "I was getting really anxious about what would happen out there." Another had just found out he tested positive for HIV. Another man cut his wrists after finding out he had been denied parole: "I just got overwhelmed by the thought of never seeing my kids until they were all grown up."

As I mention in Chapter Seven, disconnection from loved ones is a reason many prisoners give for their suicide attempts. One prisoner I interviewed made a serious suicide attempt just after hearing that his twelve-year-old daughter had been brutally raped. He was distraught about her pain and about his absolute inability to be with her in her time of need. I have spoken to many prisoners who attempted suicide after learning that a mate had gone off with someone else. Many successful suicides are motivated by jealousy.

I have talked with inmates who made serious suicide attempts because they could not stand the daily physical threats. Others—and it is almost impossible to assess how many, since most are too ashamed to talk about it—have been raped and then felt trapped in the dilemma about whether to "snitch." For still others, the thought of never holding down a job or having a family on the outside became too much to bear. Then there are the prisoners who spend almost all of their waking hours in a dark cell. They become depressed and begin to feel their situation is hopeless. The reasons in each case of prison suicide are nuanced and complex.

Prisoners suffering from psychosis and other serious mental disorders account for many prison suicides. Sometimes they kill themselves in response to "command hallucinations." These are voices that command a disturbed individual to do something, for instance to commit a violent act. When the voices command him to kill himself, the suicide risk is very high. This is because individuals suffering from severe mental disorders and responding to auditory hallucinations are unable to make sufficient contact with help-providers to listen to their advice or follow through with a commitment not to do anything self-destructive.

Even if the clinician is able, momentarily, to get the attention of such a person and arrive at some agreement not to act on suicidal impulses, as soon as the clinician has left and the voices return to command a suicidal action, the disturbed individual is very likely to disregard all prior commitments and act on the voice's orders. For example:

> I found Mr. R. A., a Native-American prisoner in his late twenties, in an administrative segregation unit. He seemed agitated, and there was a strangeness to his wide-eyed stare, a kind of strangeness I have only seen in patients suffering from acute psychosis. I asked him why he was locked in Ad Seg, and he showed me his left wrist, where there was a thick scar from a self-imposed laceration. I asked what happened and he told me the voices told him to kill himself. Mr. R. A. had been in a protected, psychiatric unit for six months, receiving high-potency antipsychotic medications, when they transferred him to this prison. "They needed the bed in the psych hospital, and I was the most dispensable patient."

There had been a delay in transferring this man's clinical chart, and he was unable to obtain his antipsychotic medications. Meanwhile, the other inmates made fun of him for "being a ding." He became progressively confused over several weeks, and then he got into a fight with a prisoner who had insulted him. He believed the guards took the other prisoner's side, and he was thrown in "the hole." By this time he had remained off his medications for three weeks. Cut off from all social contact, the voices inside his head grew louder and began to tell him "what an asshole" he was. Then they told him to kill himself. He tried to do so by slashing his wrist with a piece of metal he broke off his bed. After the suicide attempt, Mr. R. A. was sent to the infirmary for two days and had the laceration sewn up. Then "a psychiatrist came and put me back on my meds." He was charged with a disciplinary infraction for attempting suicide, and returned to Administrative Segregation.

When I met Mr. R. A., he was still hallucinating in spite of taking medications, and he had not seen a mental health professional since the psychiatrist came to see him in the infirmary and prescribed the antipsychotic medication a week prior to our interview.

## Invisible Suicides

The only reason someone commits suicide is that he cannot figure out a better alternative, given the level of his despair and the current predicament. Young people from the inner city do not believe they have many options in life. I believe this is one big reason these communities are so rife with drugs, crime, violence, and other forms of extreme risk taking. The young people do not give too much conscious thought to their future, and they do not give any serious thought to the consequences as they commit the kinds of crimes that eventually lead to their incarceration. This kind of thinking is suicidal. Inner-city gang warfare, like prison riots, involve a significant amount of unspoken suicidal inclination.

In prison, there are many ways to arrange one's own death without anyone suspecting suicide. Some prisoners do so because the self-destructive motive for their dangerous actions is unconscious. Others consciously choose to die but believe it is a sign of cowardice, or they don't want their families to live with the shame of their suicide, so they make a foolhardy escape attempt knowing the guards will shoot to kill. Or they pick a fight with a prison tough or a gang member they know will kill them. Another way a prisoner can be certain he will die is to renege on his debt to a prison drug dealer, or fail to pay a huge gambling debt.

Many successful suicides are never recorded as such because the individual dies a violent death and there are no obvious clues that a suicide has occurred. In the community, an individual might drive recklessly and get involved in a fatal crash or might shoot at the police knowing that they will shoot back. In prison, an inmate might attack a tougher prisoner, knowing very well that inmate or his buddies will retaliate and kill him. Or, he might assault an officer. Unfortunately, statistics on suicides behind bars do not include the significant number of prisoners who commit suicide by getting into a fight with a tougher prisoner or an armed guard. Many suicides go undetected and unrecorded.

## Failure to Prevent Suicide

Reports of suicides behind bars constitute an irrefutable assessment of the quality of mental health services provided to prisoners. Whereas clinicians might disagree about the diagnosis for a particular prisoner and which convicts require treatment, when a prisoner kills herself there is no argument about the fact that she should have received a more intensive and effective clinical intervention.

This is not to say that all suicides are preventable. Prisoners, on average, face a very grim future, and many tell me they are seriously contemplating suicide. A person who is really intent on killing herself might not seek treatment or mention the plan to anyone. But when a prisoner suffering from a treatable depressive episode requests help and does not receive adequate care, and then she takes her own life, her death sounds an alarm about the inadequacies of mental health care in that prison or prison system. Even if the suicidal prisoner's despair never came to the attention of the mental health staff, the large number of suicides reflects on the hopelessness bred of an increasingly harsh correctional milieu.

## Preventable Occurrences

Suicide is final. If I decide a patient is not seriously suicidal and I let him leave my office or leave the hospital, and it turns out I was wrong and he does manage to kill himself, there is no second chance to avert the tragedy.

After a suicide, it often becomes obvious in retrospect what went wrong. For example:

> A prison inmate waits until it begins to get dark on the prison yard. As the guards round up the men to return them to their cellblocks, he heads for the outer wall and begins to climb. The guard in the tower commands through the loudspeaker that he drop to the ground and put his hands up. He ignores the command and keeps climbing. The guard fires his rifle, wounding the inmate, who falls to the ground.
>
> The inmate tells the guards who descend on him with rifles drawn that he's sorry they missed—he'd rather be dead. After treatment for his wounds in the prison hospital, he is placed in solitary confinement in an Administrative Segregation unit. A psychiatrist is called to see this man in his cell. The psychiatrist interviews him briefly, noting in the chart that this inmate is a grave danger to himself and that he will return the next day to see him again. That night the prisoner hangs himself in his cell and dies.

Six months after this prisoner's death I appeared in federal court to testify about a disturbingly high incidence of serious mental illness and suicide among the inmates of that prison. The judge asked my opinion about the suicide of the prisoner who had tried to climb the wall. I told him that it seemed obvious that the treatment was grossly inadequate and that the death was preventable. The prisoner quite clearly said that he wanted to die, yet he was left in a solitary confinement cell without any suicide precautions. A psychiatrist visited him and correctly assessed the seriousness of the risk, yet the man was not transferred to a psychiatric crisis or inpatient facility. Although the psychiatrist's plan to see the prisoner the next day represented a relatively aggressive intervention for him—he rarely saw anyone more frequently than monthly—it was not an adequate treatment plan for a man who was known to be an extreme suicide risk.

The judge had already heard many suicide stories and charges of cruelty and indifference on the part of correctional staff. He asked whether, in this case, I blamed the psychiatrist. I said I believed the case reflected severe burnout in an overcrowded institution where psychiatric care was grossly inadequate. Of course, as a practitioner in the community, I would be promptly sued for malpractice were a suicide to occur after I had predicted it might yet had done nothing to prevent it. But that correctional psychiatrist probably assumed that though there was an inpatient unit in the prison, it would have been impossible to have the inmate transferred to it. There was hardly ever a bed available at the overcrowded hospital, and the admissions team had probably rejected the last five patients whom this psychiatrist had referred for emergency admission.

The more a psychiatrist cares, the more painful it is for him to supply inadequate services and turn a deaf ear to inmates' complaints. In this case, the psychiatrist probably convinced himself that he was providing the best treatment possible under the circumstances—how else would he have been able to go home at the end of the day and not lose a night's sleep? The psychiatrist was suffering from a serious case of burnout, as are many clinicians in his situation. I explained to the judge that distancing oneself from one's patients and ignoring their suffering and their needs are symptoms of burnout in public service providers. I blamed the state and the whole correctional system, since the overcrowded conditions and the lack of adequate mental health services were system-wide problems. We moved on to the next case of suicide.

In most mental health agencies in the community, as in correctional mental health programs, the "psychological autopsy" conducted after a successful suicide provides an opportunity to reassess the strengths and failings of the mental health delivery system. The mental health staff meet and go over the case, review the clinical chart, and write a report, including recommendations to improve the suicide prevention program. Alternatively, someone from the state department of corrections or the Federal Bureau of Prisons is assigned to review each suicide, and her report is sent from the central office to the staff of the prison. Ideally, the tragedy provides an important opportunity to locate and correct the program's deficiencies.

Sometimes there are a spate of suicides in a prison or prison system, and the psychological autopsies and official reviews recommend certain actions. For instance, in many systems the first action called for is more training for correctional staff in recognizing and responding to suicidal crises. The quality of the postmortem reviews varies from facility to facility. I have found that in some jails and prisons where a large number of suicides occur, the quality of the clinical charting prior to the deaths is poor and the recommendations of the psychological autopsies are not enacted in good faith. Yet I have also investigated individual prisons and prison systems where the administration and mental health staff take very seriously the occurrence of a string of suicides, and radically restructure their mental health program to better avert preventable deaths in the future.

## Just a Manipulation?

In quite a few of the completed suicides I have investigated, the staff notes from the days prior to the suicide include accusations that the prisoner is merely manipulating. I asked Mr. R. A. about manipulations, and he told me there is truth in the accusation. Sometimes he does have to say he is suicidal when he is not in order to get the attention of the psychiatrist. Remember, this is a man who is taking antipsychotic medications and hearing voices telling him to kill himself. If he has to fake a suicidal crisis in order to see the psychiatrist, just imagine how hard it is for someone who has not been diagnosed psychotic to receive help.

I reviewed a case in a California medium security prison in the early 1990s in which the prisoner stood on his bunk, tied one end of a sheet to the ceiling heater vent, stretched it taut and tied it, noose-like, around his neck. Several security officers later reported that they had walked by, seen this man standing on his bunk with a sheet suspended from the vent and tied around his neck, but did nothing because they believed "the inmate was faking a suicide attempt in order to prevent an impending transfer to Pelican Bay." Finally, the prisoner jumped from his bunk and was later found dead by hanging.

As I mention in Chapter Three, a certain number of inmates manufacture emotional symptoms hoping to be transferred to a psychiatric unit where it is easier to serve their time. It is also true that a certain number of people who attempt suicide mainly in order to get attention eventually succeed in an attempt and die. Since the incidence of suicide behind bars is high, an aggressive screening procedure is required to identify prisoners who are truly at risk. Clearly, the opinion of a security officer, who has not even received training on recognizing suicidality, about whether a seemingly suicidal inmate is merely manipulating is not an adequate assessment of suicidality.

If the staff are not sufficiently alert to the possibility of suicide and do not take seriously prisoners' "cries for help," even seriously suicidal prisoners will have to manipulate in some way if they are to get the attention they need. After reading dozens of psychological autopsies in correctional facilities in several states, I have come to the disturbing conclusion that the clinical charts of a majority of prisoners who would eventually succeed in a suicide attempt contained at least one note prior to their demise that they were "manipulating."

Suicide research aims to find the risk factors that can be noticed prior to the act, so staff can identify the high-risk cases and intervene to prevent death. In regard to prison suicide, the research is very clear. The overwhelming majority of prisoners who kill themselves are housed in solitary confinement, have a history of serious mental illness, and have made past suicide attempts. Almost as often, researchers tells us, the successful suicide had been labeled a manipulator, had just received some bad news from home, had been acting in an uncharacteristic or bizarre fashion, and had told someone he was thinking of committing suicide.

The guiding principle for mental health and security staff alike has to be: Always take prisoners' cries for help seriously until proven otherwise. But when we find that the staff are standing by as more suicides occur in solitary confinement among prisoners with a history of mental illness and prior suicide attempts, and that the staff continue to label these prisoners as manipulators and even sentence them to longer terms in lock-up for their self-destructive behaviors, we have to question whether that staff is really interested in preventing suicide.

## The Punitive Approach

Part of the problem in correctional settings is a punitive attitude that diminishes the staff's sensitivity to cues of impending suicide. It is difficult to empathize with a despairing prisoner when the staff feel he is behaving so badly that he deserves harsh punishment. For example:

> While on a tour conducted by the chief psychiatrist in a supermaximum prison unit, I asked about the suicide prevention program. The psychiatrist explained that he places prisoners who are serious suicide risks in a "quiet cell." I asked about a prisoner I had observed who was naked and lying on his back on a bed with shackles across his belly and all four limbs tied to the corners of the bed ("five-point restraints"). He reported that prisoner was considered suicidal and

> he was keeping him in restraints until he decided not to kill himself. I wrote in my report: "A psychotic or suicidal inmate would decompensate further under the stress of such treatment, and though the symptoms might temporarily disappear merely in order for the inmate to escape the treatment, the underlying psychosis or self-destructive condition is very likely to worsen."

In many prison systems a suicide attempt is treated as a disciplinary infraction and punished. Clearly, the policy of charging a prisoner who attempts to take his life with a rule violation is entirely contrary to everything we know from clinical research and practice about the assessment and treatment of suicidality.

I have found in quite a few deceased inmates' security files a posthumous citation for violating the prison rule against attempting suicide. How eerie! But this is not a rare aberration. Convicts who attempt suicide and survive must face a hearing on the charge of attempting to take their own lives, and they are likely to be sentenced to a term in solitary confinement. In addition, because the sentence is likely to include the surrendering of "good time" for days worked or for good behavior, the sentence also involves the lengthening of a prisoner's overall prison term. As a clinician, I am appalled by this widespread correctional practice. For example:

> Mr. N. M., a Mexican-American prisoner in a high-security facility in California, sent his attorney a letter on September 25, 1991, describing his suicide attempt on July 30 of that year. He had been transferred to a new, higher-security-level prison a few days prior to his suicide attempt. He had been taking relatively strong doses of antipsychotic and antidepressant medications for several years, but the psychiatrist who saw him for a brief assessment interview when he entered the new prison decided he did not need the medications and discontinued them. He complained to an MTA (medical technical assistant), who told him there was nothing he could do. Mr. N. M.

was unable to sleep without his medications, and no one listened to his complaints that he was hearing voices telling him to kill himself. A few days later, he sliced his wrist with a razor, severing a vein and narrowly missing the artery.

After the laceration was sutured in the prison hospital, he was placed on suicide watch. The medications he had been on prior to the transfer were reinstated. A few days later, he was transferred to the Administrative Segregation unit, where he was sentenced to remain for thirty days as punishment for the suicide attempt. Thirty days were also added to his prison sentence. He wrote that he felt even more suicidal after hearing the news about the lengthy sentence in solitary confinement.

The medical staff felt this inmate's complaint about voices telling him to kill himself was a "manipulation." This may have been the reason they did not send him to a psychiatric crisis unit and then, after the self-destructive act, permitted him to be punished with solitary confinement. In reality, it is unlikely that the mental health staff would have been able to prevent his removal to a lock-up unit without changes in policy and in the attitude of the security staff. But the prior discontinuation of his psychiatric medications certainly played an important role in his suicide attempt.

## The Need for Vigilance and Concern

There is no pill for suicidality. Antidepressants take several weeks to begin to work. We know that people suffering from severe depression tend not to act on their suicidal ideation until the depression begins to lift and they have the energy to follow through with the deadly plans they were mulling over while paralyzed with depression. When Prozac was released by the Food and Drug Administration for widespread prescribing, several suicides were described as side effects of the newly marketed drug. But it was not the Prozac that "caused" the suicides. Prozac was merely bringing those patients out of deep depressions, so it was proving itself effective as an antidepressant. But the patients needed to be watched, since it was already well known that suicidal people tend to act out their self-destructive impulses only after the worst of their depressive apathy is past.

Observation and talk are the only effective treatment for an acutely suicidal person. Making human contact is the crucial intervention. Medications play a secondary role. Isolation for suicidal prison inmates should be prohibited. It is possible to kill oneself in a "strip cell" or "rubber room." A prisoner who is left with no clothes and no bedding can butt her head against the wall or design an even more bizarre method of dying. Direct observation is needed if suicides are to be prevented. In a psychiatric hospital, suicidal patients are transferred to a room close enough to the nursing station for the nurses to keep an eye on them. In effective jail and prison programs, potentially suicidal inmates are placed in cells near enough to the guard's station to be observed at all times—and the guards undergo rigorous training in suicide prevention.

The policy of checking on an inmate every fifteen minutes is an acceptable second choice, *when it is done conscientiously!* I have visited prisons where notes of the every-fifteen-minute visits for an entire shift are all charted at the end of the shift. When I asked one correctional officer whether the observations actually occurred every fifteen minutes, he told me: "Not really. We get busy. I do them when I can, but often there are other fires to put out. So I just go back at the end of the day and chart one for every fifteen minutes to avoid trouble."

The risk of suicide is high in prison, and the prevention of suicide must be a high priority for prison staff. If it is to be at all successful, a prison suicide prevention program requires a conscientious staff that is not overly concerned about being manipulated and is not suffering from burnout to such an extent that they are incapable of empathizing and energetically coming to the aid of the despairing prisoner.

---

In Part II, I explored some of the features of prison life that cause prisoners unnecessary pain and suffering and tend to worsen their mental disturbances and their psychiatric disability. These features include pervasive racism, insensitivity to women's special needs, sexual harassment, rape, lack of quality visitation, and preventable suicides. Of course, time in prison is not meant to be enjoyable, but the degree of harshness and brutality that holds sway in our prisons today is not a necessary or useful part of punishment. Neither is inattention to the emotional needs of prisoners or inadequate mental health treatment for those suffering from mental disorders. Wrong-headed crime legislation and foolish correctional policies, combined with a lack of caring and outright brutality on the part of prison staff, are causing untold emotional damage to prisoners and their families, and making our streets even more dangerous.

In Part III, I present my recommendations for improving prison conditions and the plight of the mentally ill behind bars. In Chapter Nine I review how litigation can be a valuable opportunity to shine a public spotlight on some of the worst abuses and remedy some of the cruel practices that make life in prison so unbearable and psychiatric distress so severe for mentally ill prisoners. But I also discuss the limits to what litigation can accomplish, especially when courts and legislatures are bent on being ever tougher on criminals. In Chapter Ten I offer some concrete recommendations for improving correctional treatment and rehabilitation programs, but the gains from these improvements will be negligible unless we improve the way the prisons are run and revise some of our social policies and priorities. In the final chapter I review the logic of law and order that underlies some of the worst of today's correctional policies, and comment on the folly in that logic and the kind of vision that we need to change things for the better.

PART III

# An Immodest Proposal

9

# The Possibilities and Limits of Litigation

Prison litigation has improved prisoners' mental health in at least two ways: Favorable settlements and verdicts have a direct effect on prison conditions and the quality of correctional mental health services; and the experience of standing up in court as an equal adversary against those who are otherwise totally in charge of one's life in prison gives a prisoner a healthy sense of personal recourse and agency. The latter experience can serve to help alleviate what ails many prisoners in terms of emotional distress. Lawsuits brought during the last three decades have led to very concrete improvements.

Almost as soon as the prisoners began winning legal actions, politicians started calling for a reduction in prisoners' access to the courts, departments of corrections began digging in their heels to resist change, and the state and federal legislatures began devising ways to diminish prisoners' legal recourse. New laws, including the federal Prison Litigation Reform Act, have been passed to restrict prisoners' access to the courts and to limit the scope of judicial rulings regarding prison conditions. Political pressure is also put on judges who are perceived as "coddling prisoners," and some recent judicial decisions have served to undermine prisoners' successes in the courtroom. All of these developments also affect the mental health of prisoners.

## Important Gains

Court-ordered improvements in correctional mental health delivery systems result in important direct benefits. And when courts order prison systems to alleviate some of the harsh conditions, there are obvious improvements in the plight of mentally ill felons.

The indirect benefits of prison litigation are not as obvious. For instance, when an individual prisoner sues to correct an abusive practice and receives a favorable ruling, one indirect benefit is some alleviation of her sense of powerlessness and futility as a prisoner. When a group of prisoners get their day in court, one sees the pride and elevated self-esteem on their faces. Some feel less depressed, others feel less desperate and self-destructive. Finally, someone is taking their grievances seriously. The silence about harsh conditions and abusive treatment is finally broken, at least for that day in court, and the prisoners are given a voice. Contrary to skeptics who claim litigation is ineffective, I have seen big changes in the cases in which I have participated. All the horrors of contemporary prison life are not cleaned up in one fell swoop, but the improvements make a big difference in prisoners' lives.

### Class Action Lawsuits

Class action lawsuits are brought by prisoners and their advocates when their grievances are sufficiently widespread to talk about a "class." The class might be all the prisoners in an institution, all prisoners housed in a supermax unit, or all women prisoners in a state system. Sometimes a group of prisoners get together first to formulate their case and then seek outside attorneys to represent them. Sometimes, as in *Cain* v. *MDOC*, they do the case *pro se*, acting as their own attorneys.

In other cases attorneys hear from a few prisoners about an especially deplorable grievance and arrange to post notices in the prison asking whether others would like to join in a class action lawsuit. Sometimes a judge who has received a number of individual complaints from prisoners in a facility decides these cases could usefully be combined into a class action. Once a class action suit is brought, it involves all the prisoners identified as members of the class, even though relatively few of them initiated the action and became active participants. For example, in *Gates* v. *Deukmejian*, a 1989 federal class action case involving the quality of mental health services, the class included all prisoners at the California Medical Facility suffering from mental disorders.

Some of the attorneys who represent prisoners work in nonprofit prison law offices and civil rights organizations. Others are in private practice. In cases involving the possibility of a monetary settlement, the attorneys might work on a contingency basis. In many states, if the prisoners win their class action litigation, their attorneys can seek compensation from the state or federal agency being sued. In these cases, a lawyer or law firm first takes the case *pro bono*, and only attempts to recover their fees if their side prevails. And in some situations, for instance *habeus corpus* suits involving the death penalty, the courts pay attorneys to represent defendants. In other words, there are many different arrangements that make it possible for attorneys to take prison cases. But as I explain below, recent legislation and trends in case law tend to make it more difficult for prisoners to find legal counsel today. Many prisoners study in the prison law library to become "jailhouse lawyers" and represent themselves. But recent changes in prison policies limit their access to law books.

## The Impact on Mental Health

I have testified in a dozen class action lawsuits concerning the conditions of confinement and the adequacy of mental health care in jails and prisons since the mid–1970s. In each case, the issues included crowding, inadequate activities (for instance, very little out-of-cell time is permitted due to crowding and the consignment of a large number of prisoners to lock-up units), a failure to prevent suicide or rape, unfair uses of punitive segregation, and inadequate mental health care and protection from harm for prisoners known to be suffering from serious mental disorders. In every case the plaintiffs (prisoners as a class) were awarded relief, including caps on occupancy, an end to double-celling in punitive segregation units, a certain number of hours per week in an exercise area, more access to libraries, improved medical and psychiatric treatment, an end to abusive management of prisoners testing HIV-positive, and orders to employ more mental health staff and bolster treatment programs. These are significant victories.

Since crowding and idleness are known to increase the rates of violence, suicide, and emotional breakdowns in prison, court-ordered alleviation of crowding makes life much more tolerable for prisoners suffering from serious mental disorders. For instance, with less violence on the yard prisoners feel more comfortable leaving their cells and taking part in elective activities such as work assignments and athletic events. The opportunity to participate in peaceful social activities fosters more appropriate behavior and gives them an opportunity to test reality and improve social skills. Meanwhile, prisoners prone to depression are less inclined to retreat into their cells where the isolation makes their depressions worse.

The increase in friendly social connectedness and collaborative activity provides all prisoners more opportunities to talk to each other and maintain some semblance of a normal social life, which often means they will be in better shape to succeed in the community after they are released. In other words, less crowding is beneficial for the mental health of all prisoners, those suffering from mental disorders as well as those who seem relatively stable.

With the mental health services bolstered by court order, prisoners come to the attention of mental health staff more quickly when they do exhibit the signs and symptoms of significant mental disorders. The treatment they receive is more intensive, and this leads to improved coping in prison and better prognoses. In addition, with better treatment, fewer prisoners suffering from serious mental disorders are placed in punitive segregation for rule breaking and violence, and more receive the kind of treatment that is indicated for their conditions. These are only a few of the many ways that improved prison conditions and mental health services ameliorate the plight of mentally disturbed prisoners.

## Correcting Individual Wrongs

Almost every prisoner I have met has stories about all the "bum raps" they've had to bear. They tell of being "jacked up" on the street (stopped and searched by police, often roughly), and convicted of crimes they didn't commit. Even those who admit they committed the crime for which they were convicted claim that they did not have adequate legal representation. They say they have been brutalized by guards and denied their rights to visit or go to the library, they claim guards have attacked them and then written them up for "assaulting an officer," and they insist they were written up for disciplinary infractions unfairly and given excessive terms in punitive lock-up. Of course, only a fool would believe every prisoner's protestations of innocence. But some of their stories must be true. When I discover that the hearings and appeals that occur inside prisons around the country—administered by the corrections departments, not the courts—result in verdicts that go against the prisoners in over 90 percent of cases, I begin to wonder how many prisoners actually are receiving "bum raps."

Sometimes an injustice is obvious, and when the prisoner is able to get his day in court there is a redress of the grievance. Of course, the prisoner has to have the wherewithal to find a committed attorney and sustain the litigation process for a very long time. This is a gargantuan effort and few prisoners are capable of pulling it off. But when a prisoner succeeds in the effort, there are occasional rulings that renew my confidence in the legal system and make me wonder how many more prisoners are telling the truth about false charges and abuses but are denied their day in court.

Frank "Big Black" Smith's case is a clear example, both of inexcusable malice on the part of prison staff and incredible tenacity on the part of the litigants:

Frank Smith sued the state of New York for violating his civil and human rights in the wake of the prisoner uprising at Attica prison in September 1971. Mr. Smith had been a spokesperson for the prisoners during their brief takeover of the prison. After the guards regained control, they allegedly forced Mr. Smith to walk over broken glass, they struck his testicles with batons, they dropped lighted cigarettes on his body, and they played Russian roulette with a loaded gun pointed at his head. Mr. Smith, now in his mid-sixties and living in the community, testified that after the guards reestablished control of Attica prison, they forced him to lie naked on a picnic table for five hours holding a football with his chin, and told him if he let the ball roll away he would be castrated or killed.

Frank Smith is one of over a thousand Attica prisoners who filed suit in 1974, and the first to be awarded damages. On June 5, 1997, a jury found the deputy warden and the state of New York guilty of using excessive force in violation of Mr. Smith's constitutional rights, and ordered the state of New York to indemnify him in the amount of $4 million. Mr. Smith's principal attorney, Elizabeth Fink, had spent her entire career on the case.

Just imagine the difference it makes to the victim of torture when the perpetrators are found guilty by a court and restitution of some kind is ordered. At the very least, there is a beneficial effect on the degree and chronicity of posttraumatic stress disorder. But the benefits of legal redress extend far beyond those with a diagnosis of PTSD.

Mental illness, at core, involves a lack of agency, a feeling that one is not in the driver's seat in one's own life. The depressed person feels that awful things happen, and there is nothing she can do about it. The manic person believes the same thing, but defensively tries to act as though she is in complete control. The schizophrenic escapes from a reality over which he has no control into a fantasy life that at least contains some possibility of imaginary satisfaction. If, in the real world, the individual suffering from a serious and persistent mental illness is able to increase his sense of agency and to feel, in a very real sense, that he has some control over his life, there is less need to give in to depression or escape into delusion. I do not mean to imply that expensive lawsuits are justified purely for their mental health benefit—they need to evolve out of legal cause first.

In any case, opportunities for prisoners to attain a concrete legal redress of their grievances provide them an important opportunity to arrive at a modicum of mental stability. I do not know anything about Frank Smith's mental condition, but if he was a depressed ex-felon before the verdict was announced, I would guess that the judgment against his tormentors provided him cause to rise out of his depression and feel once again like he has some rights and powers as a human being.

Most lawsuits do not result in such spectacular verdicts. I am often asked to provide an opinion in a very small matter. For instance, a prisoner who is suffering from a serious mental disorder, replete with auditory hallucinations and severe paranoid delusions, is repeatedly written up by guards for talking back when they give him an order. A large law firm is asked by a local human rights group to take this man's case, and since they allocate a portion of their time to worthy *pro bono* cases, they look into the matter and decide to ask me whether I would be willing to visit the prison and assess his condition.

I interview the man and notice that he cannot cease talking long enough to let me get in a word. In my report I explain that he is suffering from a bipolar affective (or manic-depressive) disorder with psychotic features, and he is totally incapable of halting the steady stream of vituperation I began hearing as soon as I came into earshot of his cell. I speculate that each time a correctional officer approaches this prisoner he talks in the same aggressive manner, and the officers who write him up simply decide this prisoner has stepped over the line that separates permissible speech from disrespecting an officer. But, as I point out, the prisoner's disrespectful speech is a direct result of his serious mental disorder and therefore he should be seen by a psychiatrist instead of receiving disciplinary write-ups numerous enough to send him to the SHU.

In this particular case, the judge agrees with me and orders the prisoner to be removed from the SHU and to undergo psychiatric treatment. Of course, in other cases a judge is just as likely to rule that the prisoner's mental illness is no excuse for breaking prison rules—this is why so many very psychotic prisoners are housed in supermaximum security units.

I recently was asked for an opinion in a case in which a very obvious mistake was made, and a man was sent back to prison on false charges. If it had not been for the fact that the man's family hired an attorney to look into the matter, he would still be in prison.

Jed was twenty when he was convicted of illegally possessing a firearm and given a two-year fixed sentence with an additional four years on parole. When he arrived at prison, he was angry about "being sent up" and scared of being victimized. Whenever anyone acted disrespectfully toward him he made certain he took the first swing. He was involved in several fights, and in each case both participants were written up for rule violations and thrown in the hole (administrative segregation).

After a few months in prison, Jed accumulated enough rule violations to be sent to the SHU at Pelican Bay State Prison. He served the remainder of his two-year sentence in the SHU, where he remained in his cell nearly twenty-four hours a day. When his release date arrived, he was led to the front gate of the prison, given $200 "release money," and sent on his way.

When he arrived home, Jed went immediately to his old room. He emerged a few hours later and told his mother the rooms in the house seemed huge compared to the cell he'd occupied for almost two years. His mother noticed that he had lost fifty pounds in prison, and encouraged him to eat. But he did not feel like eating. He was worried about the weight loss too, and began lifting weights compulsively.

After staying up most of one night talking to her brother, Jed's twenty-year-old sister told their mother she was worried about him, "He seems in a strange mood—what if he decides to throw himself out the window, or to throw one of us out the window?" His mother was also worried. After he had been home for four days, she called his parole officer and asked whether he could help her find some counseling for her son. He told her not to worry, he would take care of everything. The next thing Jed's mother knew, the parole officer was at their door accompanied by four police officers. They arrested Jed and took him back to prison.

Jed's parole was "violated" because he was considered "mentally ill and a danger to himself and others," grounds for parole revocation in California. Shocked by this news, Jed's mother called an attorney to ask why her son was taken back to prison when he had already served his time and had not broken any laws since his release.

The correctional psychiatrist assigned to evaluate Jed began by informing Jed that the interview was entirely voluntary and there would be no confidentiality. Jed was angry about being sent back to prison, and decided he did not want to say much to the psychiatrist under the circumstances. So he ended the psychiatric examination after fifteen minutes.

The psychiatrist did not get much information from the interview. But in his report to the parole board, he wrote that Jed had threatened to kill himself or his mother or sister and that he was hearing voices during the four days he was at home. He admitted that during the interview there was no "gross evidence of a psychosis" and that Jed "did not appear to be responding to internal stimuli" and "did not state any specific suicidal or violent ideation." But because the parole officer had reported that Jed was hearing voices and threatening to throw someone out the window, he assigned Jed the diagnosis "psychotic disorder, not otherwise specified," and opined that Jed posed a danger to himself and others. Based on that diagnosis, the parole board decided to keep Jed in prison for one additional year, most of it to be spent in solitary confinement.

> I examined Jed a few months later and did not detect any signs or symptoms of psychosis. Jed explained he had stayed in his room when he returned home because, after two years in the SHU, he was not ready to relate to people. He had planned to come out of his room gradually, when he felt safe. He never heard any imaginary voices and denied threatening suicide or violence. I checked with his mother, and it turned out his sister had merely imagined that he might be dangerous, but Jed had never said anything to her about throwing himself or her out the window. Once Jed returned to prison, he decided not to speak to the psychiatrists but instead to wait for a legal proceeding to free him.
>
> I was impressed by the soundness of his strategizing and his ability to control the wrath he felt about being falsely re-imprisoned after having served his time. I don't believe the parole board would have considered my professional opinion had his lawyer not sued the state to release him. But in any case, he was released as soon as the department of corrections realized the violation of his parole had been based on factual errors and the examining psychiatrist's very incorrect assumption that any prisoner who refused to talk to him, even after he announced the interview was voluntary, must be paranoid and psychotic.

Jed was only able to fight a wrong decision by the parole board and prevail because his mother hired an attorney to represent him. There are a huge number of cases in which a prisoner is wrongly imprisoned and isn't able to gain legal representation. And the trend toward harsher sentences and an end to "coddling" is resulting in prisoners having even less access to legal representation and to the courts today.

## Giving Prisoners a Voice

It is always inspiring to see people who have been treated shabbily stand up and demand their rights, as prisoners are doing in court. Inside the prisons, felons have little or no power. They are harshly punished for saying anything that a correctional officer might interpret as disrespectful. They lose over 90 percent of hearings on the merit of their claims that they are being punished unfairly. When they appear before a parole board and receive a negative decision, they have very little right to appeal. But when their legal complaints are certified as valid by a court of law and they appear as plaintiffs in civil lawsuits, their standing in court is equal to the standing of the defendants, including the warden and the director of corrections.

This simple benefit of access to the courts was explained to me by a man I interviewed recently who had "maxed out of the SHU" at the state correctional institution (SCI) at Greene in Pennsylvania. He had been in near-solitary confinement for eighteen months until his fixed sentence ran out and he was released. He had barely graduated high school. I asked him how he managed to maintain his sanity while watching prisoners in nearby cells go crazy and begin shouting at all hours of the night and throwing excrement. He responded: "I sued them [the state]. I ordered law books and read them, and whenever they did something illegal I filed suit. I never won any of the cases—a couple of them did go to trial—but the process of learning enough law to stand up for myself kept me from 'bugging out' all those months I was by myself in that dreary cell."

I witnessed a similar phenomenon when I testified in *Cain* v. *Michigan Department of Corrections* (MDOC). At a time when corrections departments are rationalizing endless restrictions on prisoners' freedoms as security measures, and federal courts are refusing to intervene, eight prisoners acting *in pro se* (as their own attorneys) in Michigan State Court on behalf of 41,000 men and 2,000 women prisoners, with attorneys collaborating in the case, launched a class action lawsuit ten years ago. The case finally went to trial in April 1997, and because the state court judge is unusual in his willingness to permit the prisoners to put on far-ranging evidence as long as they can prove it is relevant, the trial is likely to continue for quite some time.

The courtroom in *Cain* v. *MDOC* is a gymnasium in a local jail near Jackson with tables for the judge, the lawyers, and the witnesses, plus rows of benches for the press and audience. Over a dozen men and women prisoners arrive in shackles to sit at the plaintiff's table. I testified about the detrimental effects that the proposed restrictive policy—limiting the number of possessions prisoners can keep in their cells and requiring them to wear uniforms—would probably have on the mental health of prisoners. For instance, my research demonstrated that many prisoners in lower security prisons would refuse visits if they were forced to wear prison uniforms, and the lack of contact with loved ones would negatively affect their mental health and ultimately lead some of them to attempt suicide.

The prisoner/paralegal who prepared me to testify and conducted my direct and cross-examination in court never graduated from college. Yet he is known in prison litigation circles as a brilliant, creative legal strategist. And he feels confident facing an assistant attorney general in court.

*Cain* v. *MDOC* is still in process. How the judge will eventually rule is unclear. But the prisoners win little victories on a regular basis. For example, the supermaximum security unit in Michigan's prison system, located in Ionia, is called Ionia Max or I-Max. State correctional policy prohibits the placement of mentally disturbed prisoners in I-Max. The prisoner/litigants put one prisoner on the stand who was housed at I-Max. He testified that he had taken antipsychotic medications for years, but a prison psychiatrist discontinued his prescriptions a few months before he received the disciplinary write-up that resulted in his transfer to I-Max.

He did not know why his medications were discontinued but complained that without them he became delusional and was unable to control the angry outbursts that caused the guards to write him up. The prisoners won their point: Even though the policy states that mentally disordered prisoners are not to be housed in supermaximum security, it is very easy for the staff to take prisoners off their psychiatric medications, declare their mental illness resolved, and send them to a supermaximum security unit. The prisoners sitting at the plaintiff's table were very proud of getting this noted in the court record. The testimony may not lead to a specific court ruling, but the fact that the practice of taking mental patients off their medications before sending them to solitary confinement can be litigated serves notice to the state that their correctional policies can be exposed in a courtroom.

## Ending the Secrecy, Breaking the Silence

We know from history and research on institutional dynamics that keepers with absolute power tend to act cruelly toward the kept. This is especially true if there is no outside surveillance. When a nation's "secret police" torture their prisoners, secrecy surrounds the entire procedure. The press are not permitted access to the police stations and jails, and the prisoners are silenced. Quite a few cases have come to light in the United States in recent decades in which police internal affairs divisions and departmental review boards fail to uncover specific acts of brutality and wrongful deaths perpetrated by members of the force. An independent investigator or citizen's review board eventually discovers sufficient evidence of criminal misconduct to force the local prosecutor or the U.S. Department of Justice to step in and take the offending officers to court to answer for their crimes.

We know from historical precedents, such as the prisoner-lease practices of the post–Civil War South, that once prisoners are out of sight and mind they can be treated horribly, in many cases as if they were chattel. I have mentioned several instances of obvious cruelty and criminal misconduct on the part of correctional officers, including gladiatorial battles staged by guards at Corcoran State Prison and the forced dunking of Vinson in a scorching bath at Pelican Bay State Prison. Imagine the harm to the mental health of prisoners! Yet these unfathomable abuses of prisoners were taken seriously by state officials only after they leaked into newspaper headlines and television newscasts.

In this light, it is very upsetting to realize that legislatures and correctional authorities are instituting a growing number of restrictions on media and public access to the prisons. For instance, "gag orders" have been issued in several states. The California legislature recently passed a law forbidding journalists access to prisoners without the prior approval of the department of corrections. In practice this means no interviews are permitted with prisoners, unless the department of corrections wants to parade a prisoner in front of a press conference to dispel public concerns about brutal correctional practices. But this law also means that the same officials who are under federal indictment for their role in the deaths that occurred at Corcoran State Prison control press access to prisoners who witnessed the fights and shootings. Secrecy is the theme, as if lawmakers and correctional administrators are trying to accomplish damage-control by limiting public revelations about the abuses that occur behind bars.

Prison litigation plays a key role in breaking the silence. Outsiders gain access to prisons only with great difficulty. Visitors might hear about horrible conditions and abuses from the prisoners they visit, but they cannot observe them firsthand. Most of my tours of prisons have been ordered by courts. The prisoners bring suit as a class, attorneys enter the case, the court orders the prison system to permit the plaintiffs sufficient access to conduct their case, and the plaintiffs bring their experts into the prisons to evaluate conditions and practices.

When I ask to see a clinical chart or the report of a "psychological autopsy," the prison is required to show them to me. When I ask to tour a particular unit of the prison, or interview a particular prisoner or staff member, the warden is under court order to permit access. This gives experts in litigation quite a unique opportunity to determine what is actually occurring in correctional institutions today.

Court proceedings go on the public record. Anything that is disclosed in court, as long as the judge does not restrict public access, is available for public broadcast. This is not to say that the press comes to court in great numbers to find out what is going on behind bars. The courtrooms where I have testified have been relatively empty. Occasionally a newspaper reporter or a television news crew drops in, but few remain there long enough to get the full story. Still, court proceeding give a rare opportunity to make the truth available to the public. Of course, getting the public to care about the plight of prisoners is another matter.

High-profile class action lawsuits break the near-total secrecy that usually surrounds daily life in the prisons. After being forced into the bath that burned his skin off, Vinson sued the state of California. A large class action lawsuit, *Madrid* v. *Gomez*, involving the same unit at Pelican Bay State Prison, resulted in a federal judge declaring that a supermaximum security unit is no place to house mentally ill prisoners. In each case, there were headlines, and the public had a rare opportunity to find out what is really going on inside our prisons. Again, the indirect effect on prisoners' mental health included an ending of the silence and some degree of renewed hope that someone cares about the way they are being treated.

## It Is Possible to Implement Rulings

Some critics of legal remedies for prison problems argue that a prison system can resist court orders and consent decrees indefinitely, and therefore lawsuits are doomed to failure. Although it is true that the states and federal government can dig in their heels and prevent meaningful prison reform, it is also true that more reasonable prison authorities can accept court mandates and make remarkable changes in the way they approach prisoners.

For example, I observed the power of administrations to halt cruel and inhuman punishments when I toured Indiana's Maximum Control Facility (MCF) in Westville in July 1997. Prisoners at the MCF, a majority of whom were people of color, sued the state a few years after the unit opened in 1991, claiming the harsh conditions and the brutality of the guards violated their civil rights and constituted cruel and unusual punishment. Prior to the lawsuit, the prisoners had been complaining for weeks about the consistently poor quality of the food.

> One day the prisoners in the MCF were served cold hamburgers for lunch. Several prisoners picked apart the patties and found hairs and grit mixed in with the poor quality meat. The guards who were serving the food were unresponsive to their complaints. A couple of prisoners on the unit decided to retain their food trays with the uneaten hamburgers to show the shift commander why they were refusing to eat.
>
> The guards were angered by the refusal, and began immediately to make rounds of the entire pod, asking each prisoner if he was going to return his food tray. Several prisoners said, "Not until I get to talk to the commander about the poor quality of this hamburger." The guards immediately bellowed: "That's a refusal!" Not another word was spoken. The guards left the section and formed a cell extraction team. The next thing the prisoners knew, five large officers in riot gear barged into their cells and removed them, one at a time. Quite a few prisoners had to be taken to the infirmary for treatment of their injuries.
>
> At that time it was not unusual for two or three cell extractions to be conducted per day at the MCF. The prisoners' lawsuit and a Human Rights Watch investigation uncovered incidents in which officers repeatedly teamed up to beat prisoners and then charge them with "assaulting an officer."
>
> The prisoners' class action lawsuit was settled in February 1994 with the signing of an Agreed Entry (a pretrial settlement agreement). Changes were instituted. For instance, the superintendent of the MCF was replaced. The new superintendent, attempting to comply with the Agreed Entry's ban on senseless beatings and cell extractions, instituted a policy requiring officers to give prisoners several opportunities to change their minds before initiating an extraction. He also

> required officers to summon the shift commander to the cell to try to convince a recalcitrant prisoner to comply with orders, and stipulated that the superintendent himself must then be contacted prior to the commencement of a cell extraction. At the very least, the new policy effected a "cooling off period" for the officers as well as the prisoners. The result was a sudden and massive decrease in the number of cell extractions at the MCF.

If the Indiana Department of Corrections can dramatically reduce the number of cell extractions in a supermaximum facility simply by rewriting the policy for initiating extractions, other states can also cut down on the frequency of brutality against prisoners, improve conditions, and upgrade the quality of mental health services in the prisons—if they choose to do so. But if they choose to block the courts' efforts to guarantee the constitutional rights of prisoners, the sad truth is they are all too able to do that as well.

## One Step Forward, Two Steps Back

Lawsuits are difficult to organize and expensive to bring. They can create hostilities among the parties, causing the defendants (usually a state or federal prison administration) to dig in their heels and resist the court-ordered improvements. This is a time of conservative hegemony and widespread support for the law-and-order approach to criminal justice issues. Even when legal battles direct the public's attention to the hardships and abuses suffered by prisoners, politicians and legislatures are not very likely to support or even explore the possibility of prison reform. They are too busy cutting budgets to seriously consider spending more money on reforms the public is not demanding.

Laws are passed aimed at limiting the courts' ability to order prison reform. Judges who permit the prisoners their day in court and rule in their favor are attacked by conservative politicians for "coddling prisoners." In many cases the progress that prisoners had been making in the courts is halted, and the earlier gains in terms of mental health benefits are reversed.

## The State Digs in Its Heels

Although prison litigation can accomplish quite a lot of good, the legal process is not very effective at fine-tuning the renovation of prison systems. Legal battles set up advocacy situations that starkly polarize the sides. For instance, when the prisoners charge that the prison system is violating their constitutional rights, the prison system defends its practices, often becoming less flexible in the process. Even though the plaintiffs may win on the large issues, there is insufficient good will after the trial for the state or federal government to carry through with the kinds of flexible approaches that would be needed to really improve the plight of prisoners. Later, when the prisoners' attorneys complain that the government is not following through with the mandated changes, the courts bow out of the dispute, saying they are not willing to micromanage the improvement of state or federal prison systems. Meanwhile, the departments of corrections, reeling from the legal defeat, are unwilling to make any improvements except what the court has specifically ordered. Too often a stand-off results, leading to very little cooperation between the prisoners' advocates and the defenders of the prison system.

## The Shell Game

The states and the federal prison systems can resist change in many ways. For example, one of the easiest ways for a prison system to block prisoners' ability to gain relief from the courts is to wait until the lawsuit is brought and then transfer the problem or the abusive practice that inspired the lawsuit to another prison, one that is not covered by the lawsuit or the court's jurisdiction. This kind of clever, cynical maneuver reminds me of the shell game. The operator of the shell game moves the walnut shells around so fast that the observer never guesses which one covers the coin. Similarly, when prison administrators wish to defy the spirit of the law against cruel and unusual punishment, they can move prisoners and programs around so that they never have to comply with large sections of a court order.

I observed this ploy for the first time in the *Toussaint* v. *Enomoto* case. The prisoners as a class sued the California Department of Corrections, claiming that double-celling prisoners in Security Housing Units (at that time SHUs were located at San Quentin and Folsom Prisons—Pelican Bay and Corcoran had not been built), where they were confined to their cells nearly twenty-four hours each day, constituted cruel and unusual punishment. Psychiatric concerns were intricately involved in the case. For instance, the crowding had negative effects on prisoners' mental health, and mentally ill prisoners in these units were subject to victimization. The federal judge ruled in the prisoners' favor, ordering that prisoners in the SHUs of both institutions had to be placed in single cells.

While the class action lawsuit was in process, the state built a new prison adjacent to Folsom Prison. At first, "Old Folsom" and "New Folsom" were both directed by the same warden, but they were declared separate administrative units by the department of corrections. A lock-up unit was established at New Folsom, and prisoners were double-celled within it. When the prisoners' attorneys complained that double-celling prisoners in the lock-up units at New Folsom violated the judge's order in the Toussaint case, the state replied that since New Folsom was a separate entity, the judge's order did not cover its lock-up units. Although the ruling in Toussaint stood up to appeals, the state's claim that New Folsom was not covered by the ruling also stood up. The state lost the lawsuit, but continued to double cell very dangerous prisoners in some of the highest security lock-up units that existed at that time.

I witnessed this kind of maneuver again in the case of *Gates* v. *Deukmejian*. Mentally ill prisoners as a class sued the state of California, claiming that the care provided to the mentally disordered prisoners housed at the California Medical Facility (CMF) at Vacaville was entirely inadequate. The federal judge would eventually agree with the prisoners and order the state to upgrade the mental health services at that facility. But before the legal case had proceeded very far, the state transferred approximately 500 of the 1,300 prisoners who had been classified as mentally ill out of CMF and sent them to other prisons around the state. The attorneys for the prisoners protested that these 500 prisoners were "part of the class" and could not be transferred out of CMF while the Gates case was in process. On that point, the plaintiffs (prisoners) lost.

The state claimed that although those 500 prisoners had suffered from mental illnesses in the past, their psychiatrists decided (after the lawsuit had commenced) that they were sufficiently recovered to go to nontreatment facilities. Of course, the department of corrections had merely transferred the men who seemed relatively stable at one point in time. Many of them were suffering from serious and long-term mental illnesses and would experience exacerbations and repeated breakdowns in the prisons to which they were transferred, where few mental health services were available.

I will mention one further example of the shell game. In Indiana, part of the cause of action in the lawsuit involving the supermaximum MCF was the housing of severely mentally disordered inmates in a segregation unit where the harsh conditions would probably worsen their emotional disturbances. As part of the Agreed Entry that ended the lawsuit, the state agreed not to house mentally disordered prisoners at the MCF. But soon thereafter a large number of mentally ill prisoners showed up at the state's newer supermaximum facility, the SHU at Wabash Valley Correctional Institution in Carlisle, which was not covered by the lawsuit at the MCF.

In other words, the agreement that ends a legal action is only as solid as the good will of the signatories.

## The Prison Litigation Reform Act

On April 27, 1996, President Clinton signed the Prison Litigation Reform Act (PLRF), a piece of legislation that was designed to restrict prisoners' access to federal courts and to limit the courts' ability to remedy constitutional violations. The Act limits the time a court-approved consent decree will be in effect, in most cases placing a limit of two years. This is a big blow to prisoners and their attorneys, since it takes many years to mount a large class action lawsuit, and the state can stall the implementation process by waiting months or years to make changes. With a two-year cap on the life of the consent decree, some of the law firms that finance the class actions will decide that the large lawsuits are no longer worth bringing. The PLRA also sets strict limits on the kinds of relief that a court can order and the fees it can order paid to the prisoners' attorneys. And it ends long-standing waivers on court costs for indigent prisoners and requires all prisoners to pay large fees prior to filing.

So far, the PLRA is accomplishing what it was designed for: The number of prisoner *habeus corpus* appeals and the number of prisoner civil rights filings has declined significantly since the President signed the PLRA.

## The Courts Back Off

Public opinion shapes judicial decisions. Between the 1960s and the 1980s, courts rendered opinions that assumed prisoners have specific constitutional rights that must be respected. Since the early 1990s, although stopping short of denying that prisoners have rights, courts have been retreating to more limited rulings, as though they believe the judiciary should not make very strenuous efforts to correct prison policies that violate prisoners' rights. Several federal courts have recently rendered adverse decisions in prisoners' class action suits, arguing that the courts should not be telling states and their departments of corrections how to run the prisons. Other courts have ruled that relatively harsh punishments are acceptable as long as the states can prove they are necessary for security purposes. Of course, this trend has negative ramifications for mentally ill prisoners. The courts are less likely than they were a decade ago to order prison systems to ameliorate harsh conditions and improve mental health services.

The way the courts address the issue of prison rehabilitation illustrates the ultimate limitations of litigation. I am often told by attorneys for the prisoners to avoid the topic of rehabilitation when I testify in court. I ask why, and they tell me that there is no constitutional requirement that departments of corrections supply prisoners with opportunities to rehabilitate themselves. How sad, I think to myself, but as I take the stand I make a mental note not to exhibit too much enthusiasm about the project of rehabilitating prisoners lest the state's attorneys general use my unrealistic recommendations to impeach my entire testimony. In Chapter Ten I explain the relevance of education and rehabilitation programs to the mental health of prisoners, but obviously it will take more than litigation to establish adequate programs.

The legal system was not designed to echo public opinion. In fact, the United States Constitution requires the courts to maintain their separateness from government and, by implication, from politics and public opinion polls. The courts have a responsibility to stand against the popular sensibility of "lock 'em up and throw away the key" wherever that sensibility leads to correctional policies that violate prisoners' constitutional and human rights. But in an age when the "law-and-order" sensibility enjoys widespread currency, every judge who has to face reelection must think twice before rendering any decision the public might consider "soft on crime."

One of the arguments made by those who want to limit prisoners' access to the courts is that they bring "frivolous suits," and taxpayers should not have to pay for their access to the courts when all they want is to turn the prisons into resorts. In fact, occasionally there is a "frivolous" lawsuit. But the number of very worthy legal actions brought by prisoners, such as the ones I have mentioned, far outnumber the frivolous ones. It is very appropriate for the courts of a democratic society to consider worthy issues raised by prisoners. The conditions in most prisons today are truly cruel and inhuman, the mental health services are grossly inadequate, and the abuses of prisoners are widespread. Prisoners suffer severe emotional distress from unnecessary hardships, and this is an issue the courts should be examining closely.

---

Prison reform litigation has definitely brought about important improvements in prison conditions and the quality of mental health services behind bars. As a result, 430 prisons in the United States are currently under some form of consent decree or injunction concerning the conditions of confinement and the adequacy of health and mental health services.

But recent legislation and judicial decisions are making a legal strategy for bringing about prison reform much more problematic. Though litigation is still worth pursuing, other strategies are sorely needed. In the next chapter, I outline some of the changes I envision in terms of conditions of confinement, mental health treatment, and rehabilitation. I also outline some of the changes in the entire criminal justice system that will be needed if substantial improvements in mental health services are to be effected.

# 10

# Recommendations for Treatment and Rehabilitation

I can't end this book without making recommendations about how to fix what I have pointed out is terribly wrong in our prisons, especially regarding mentally disordered prisoners. But recommendations at what level? Would it suffice to say that we need to double or perhaps even quadruple the number of psychiatrists employed in the prisons? Yes, that would help a little. More seriously disturbed prisoners would be seen and staff could spend a little more time talking with them. But that would not alter the fact that many psychiatric patients are victimized and many others wind up in punitive detention. Medicating a prisoner who must remain in his cell all day is totally unacceptable mental health treatment, and ultimately it causes worse mental disorders and creates immense public danger.

The history of imprisonment tends to follow a cyclic pattern. First, in reaction to the horrors and abuses of a period of cruel punishment, there is a wave of prison reform, replete with optimistic claims for rehabilitating criminals. After a while, due to inattention or perhaps a waning of sympathy for lawbreakers during a time of economic insecurity, there is deterioration of prison conditions and demolition of the programs that had been touted for their rehabilitative potential. Suddenly these programs are deemed ineffectual, or stigmatized as "coddling prisoners." There follows a period of harsh authoritarian control in the prisons, accompanied by a significant amount of unchecked sadism on the part of guards. Abuses of prisoners proliferate. Eventually a line is crossed in terms of what decent citizens will tolerate, the whistle is blown, and there are sensational headlines and public outrage once again, leading to new calls for reform.

The quality of prison mental health programming tends to fluctuate with public attitudes about rehabilitation in general. When educational and vocational training programs are cut and most of the prisoners are idle, the mental health treatment program is certain to be grossly underfunded and essentially limited to prescribing medications for disturbed prisoners. When rehabilitation in general is a priority within corrections systems, psychiatric treatment and rehabilitation efforts blossom and prisoners with psychiatric disorders are supported in their efforts to make use of all available treatment and rehab programs.

In other words, where the goal of corrections is "to correct" or to rehabilitate the offender, adequate mental health care is viewed as a necessary ingredient in the larger rehabilitative project. On the other side of the cycle, when harsh punishment is the sole aim of incarceration—and this is very much the case today—there is less faith in the rehabilitative possibilities of imprisonment in general and less attention to the treatment needs of prisoners suffering from serious and long-term mental disorders.

We are at the point today at which harshness and brutality within the prisons have proliferated and the public is just becoming aware of the extent of the cruelty. It's a good time to make recommendations for positive change.

---

My recommendations for improving mental health services inside prisons and resolving the mental health crisis include changes on three levels:

1. Correctional mental health services and psychiatric rehabilitation programs must be upgraded. I outline ten essential components of the upgrade below.
2. We need to change the prisons as institutions, including revitalizing general rehabilitation programs and ending the use of supermaximum security units.
3. Finally, changes are needed at a societal level. We have to put an end to prison crowding and racial disparities in sentencing. We need to stop sending nonviolent drug offenders and mentally disordered felons onto prison yards with murderers and rapists, and we need to upgrade the public mental health system substantially.

I'll mention some existing model programs in the United States and worldwide that demonstrate that a better approach to imprisonment is possible. The fate of mentally ill prisoners depends on our commitment as a society to envision and enact better ways to achieve criminal justice.

## Ten Essentials of a Mental Health Program

We can begin with the six components of a minimally adequate correctional mental health treatment program formulated by the federal district court in *Ruiz* v. *Estelle* in 1980, including a systematic screening procedure and treatment that entails more than segregation and involves a sufficient number of mental health professionals to provide adequate services to all prisoners suffering from serious mental disorders (see Minimum Standards of Care in Chapter Three).

But this formulation in its original form is far from adequate. For example, prisoners suffering from "major mental illnesses" are not the only ones who need treatment. Prisoners with substance abuse problems and those who are experiencing flashbacks and panic attacks following a rape also need quality mental health services. So I'll embellish and expand upon the six components identified in Ruiz while enlarging the list to ten.

What I believe the courts should be calling for is a system that provides the following:

## 1. Comprehensive Levels of Care

Mental health systems are just that, systems. There need to be inpatient psychiatric wards, outpatient clinics, emergency services, day treatment programs, case management, halfway houses, supported living in the community, vocational training programs, and so forth. Similarly, correctional mental health services need to involve a comprehensive system if we are to do better than medicating prisoners and warehousing them in their cells.

There are minimum standards for correctional health care, published by the National Commission on Correctional Health Care, the American Psychiatric Association, and the American Public Health Association. The National Commission on Correctional Health Care inspects and accredits prisons and correctional systems that comply with its standards. But the standards tend to be very abstract. An example is this statement from the 1997 edition of the National Commission's standards: "Written policy and defined procedures require, and actual practice evidences, that the prison has written arrangements for providing hospital and specialized ambulatory care for medical and mental illnesses in facilities that meet state licensure requirements for hospital care."

In practice, who is to say that all the prisoners who need hospitalization and outpatient care receive it? I have discovered many seriously disturbed prisoners languishing in their cells without adequate psychiatric treatment in prisons that received accreditation. Just as no legal procedure can guarantee adequate mental health care, no accrediting system is foolproof. At the present time, prison systems are not required by state or federal law to achieve accreditation. A positive first step toward improving correctional mental health services would be to require all prison systems to meet the minimum standards and achieve the accreditations that currently exist.

Prison systems are not required to provide extensive "talking therapy" or prolonged stays in restful hospital settings. These are luxuries reserved for those who can afford them. But just as the homeless person in the community who hallucinates is entitled to a thorough psychiatric examination, medications when appropriate, admission to a county hospital if necessary, and case management to maximize his functioning—so is a prisoner who suffers from a serious mental disturbance entitled to a variety of services aimed at minimizing his immediate suffering as well as his long-term disability.

Most of the systems I have toured contain an inpatient psychiatric ward or contract with a nearby hospital or university medical center to provide inpatient care. But there are problems in many prisons, including a relative shortage of beds, an excessively short length of hospital stay, and a lack of authority on the part of the mental health staff within the prisons to admit the prisoners they believe require inpatient care.

I recommend "direct admitting privileges" for psychiatrists who work in the prisons. In other words, when a psychiatrist working in a lock-up unit or a general population prison discovers an acutely psychotic or suicidal patient she believes needs to be admitted to a hospital, she can write an order and have the patient admitted without the need for a second evaluation at the hospital gate by the admissions team. In addition, procedures need to be in place that guarantee no prisoner who needs to be admitted will be refused because of insufficient bed space. Of course, each prison system has its own unique set of problems to work out.

Prisoners who suffer emotional breakdowns sufficiently serious as to require psychiatric hospitalization will most likely need to be sent to some kind of protected or supported correctional setting after they are discharged. Lacking a supportive setting and left to their own devices, they are very likely to get into trouble as victims or as rule-breakers. Many quit taking their prescribed medications and suffer relapses. These mentally disturbed prisoners need intermediate treatment programs, places where they are somewhat protected from danger and supported in their efforts to understand their mental illnesses and the reasons they need to comply with the treatment. And they need to be involved in meaningful, supervised social activities such as group counseling sessions, school classes, vocational training, and supervised recreation.

I have mentioned other services that mentally ill prisoners need. For instance, they need case managers to keep track of their whereabouts in the prison system and to make certain they stay out of harm's way and participate in the kinds of programs that are likely to help them maintain emotional stability. They need adequate medication management with a psychiatrist who will spend sufficient time talking to them, take seriously their complaints about side effects of medications, monitor blood chemistry levels, and make adequate notes in their charts. An adequate number of social workers with small enough caseloads must be available to talk to a prisoner's family and make a home visit in an emergency, for instance when a prisoner's spouse or child is in serious trouble and the prisoner's mental deterioration results from a lack of contact. There need to be a wide variety of treatment modalities within the prisons so that prisoners with different needs and disabilities can be offered the services they need.

## 2. Suicide Prevention

We know how to prevent suicides. The critical ingredients are staff training, a high degree of vigilance, arrangements for direct observation, and adequate treatment programs for prisoners who present an imminent risk. Often the prisoner who is contemplating suicide is not in treatment. Correctional staff can be trained to watch for the clues and to act effectively to prevent suicide.

Once a prisoner is recognized as a serious suicide risk, she should be seen by a mental health professional and precautions must be instituted to be reasonably certain she will not take her own life. We know what not to do. She should not be placed in solitary confinement. Constant surveillance is an essential component of treatment.

Medications might be indicated, for instance an antipsychotic medication for a delusional prisoner who hears voices commanding him to take his own life. As I mention in Chapter Eight, antidepressant medications require a few weeks to take effect, so it is entirely unacceptable for a psychiatrist to visit a suicidal prisoner at his cell door and merely prescribe an antidepressant.

The prisoner needs someone to talk to, in depth, to find out what is behind the profound despair. A sensitive intervention provides the prisoner a sense that someone cares and will try to help. Above all else, there needs to be a resolve on the part of correctional administrators, staff, and mental health clinicians to put a rigorous suicide prevention program in place.

## 3. Group Therapy and Special Problems

Group therapy is essential for prisoners suffering from serious mental disorders, including but not limited to groups that focus on the need for mentally disordered prisoners to understand their conditions and comply with their medication regimens.

In addition, group therapy and counseling focused on specific problems—including substance abuse, domestic violence, and parenting issues—have proven very effective with a much larger group of felons in prison. Yet in most of the prisons I have toured there are relatively few groups in progress. The psychiatrists explain they are too busy prescribing medications to conduct groups and the psychologists say they spend most of their time writing reports for courts and parole boards. Many members of the mental health staff complain that they are not sufficiently trained in group process.

Community drug and alcohol treatment programs have progressed quite a lot in recent years, and outcome studies show they succeed in helping a large number of people stay clean and sober. There are reports of substance abuse treatment programs that are successful in jails and prisons, but relatively few prison systems provide serious educational and therapeutic programs to felons with histories of drug and alcohol abuse. Experts in the field of substance abuse should be brought into the prisons to train the staff and set up state-of-the-art programs aimed at decreasing the likelihood that prisoners will return to their old addictions once they are released.

Similarly, we know from outcome studies that well-conducted educational and therapeutic groups serve to reduce recidivism in perpetrators of domestic violence and sexual assault. I am not saying that people convicted of these violent crimes should be excused because of a mental disorder, nor should they be "coddled." But neither should they be left to serve their time without any opportunity to mend their ways. However serious their crimes, leaving them to suffer the traumas of prison life with no opportunity to work on their issues will make it more likely they will reoffend after they get out. Alternatively, offering them a serious group counseling program run by experts on their problem will significantly decrease the chances of their reoffending. We know that there are some men whose proclivity for violence will not be affected, but consider all the cases in which such an intervention will make a difference.

Correctional programs to retrain men to express themselves and work out differences without resorting to violence are often token, at best. For instance, in many states judges include in a sentence for domestic violence or sexual assault the stipulation that the convict is to undergo treatment prior to release from prison. In many overcrowded prisons the mandated treatment is left until the last year of the man's term. This means that the man will be influenced by the prison culture for most of his term, which will probably intensify his rage and only teach him to strike out more violently, and then in his last year of incarceration he will be placed in a group therapy for batterers or sex offenders in preparation for release. Is it any wonder that these groups often fail? Rather, the interventions that are most successful in ending men's violence in the community should be brought into the jails and prisons, on a preventive basis, for all inmates prone to these crimes, during the entirety of their stays in correctional settings.

Mental health treatment is also needed for the survivors of violent crime—and there are many survivors in prison. Consider the female survivor of childhood molestation and domestic violence during adulthood. Group counseling is known to be very effective in bolstering women's self-esteem, helping them work through past traumas, and encouraging them to make better choices when they leave prison. Groups for male survivors can accomplish as much.

A therapeutic program can help the prison rape victim cope with the aftereffects of that horrendous trauma. Such a program could be modeled on successful rape and domestic abuse treatment programs in the community. For instance, security and mental health staff could be trained in the art of providing a safe place for the victim to heal. At the very least they could be taught why they should avoid replaying the trauma by forcing the victim to identify the perpetrator or sending her to punitive detention. Prisoners who suffer from the symptoms of PTSD need a trusting therapeutic relationship within which they can begin to work through the trauma of rape or the multiple traumas they have experienced throughout their lives.

Other kinds of groups are needed as well. For instance, anger management groups can be very effective, as can groups designed to help prisoners understand their role as parents and work through their grief about being separated from their loved ones. Group counseling can help prisoners who are HIV-positive or suffer from AIDS work through their grief and come to grips with their predicament. Group experiences, whether designed as therapy or psycho-education, provide willing prisoners with an important alternative to the isolation that otherwise dominates prison life.

## 4. Psychiatric Rehabilitation Programs

The emphasis in public mental health programs has shifted from a psychotherapy/treatment model to a psychiatric rehabilitation model. The thinking is that psychotherapy is relatively expensive and ineffective with severely disturbed and substance-abusing people. Instead of offering the people suffering from serious and persistent mental disorders long-term therapy, outpatient clinics are being closed and resources are being shifted to day treatment, halfway houses, supported independent living, vocational training, and case management—the main components of modern psychiatric rehab.

Psychiatric rehabilitation focuses on clients' goals and downplays the specifics of their psychopathology. Instead of encouraging psychiatrically disabled people to explore their childhood traumas and inner conflicts, psychiatric rehabilitation aims to help them "live, learn, and work" in community environments of their choosing. The emphasis is on "the skills of daily living," including medication compliance and avoidance of illicit drugs, alcohol, and criminal activities. The case manager coordinates a client's community care services and tracks her progress and whereabouts.

This kind of thinking and programming can usefully be translated into what I term "intermediate level" correctional mental health services. And in many correctional settings, this is being done. Instead of discharging a prisoner from a psychiatric inpatient ward right back out into the general population, certain tiers or cellblocks can be designated as intermediate psychiatric care facilities, and the prisoners within them can be supervised in their daily activities until they learn to get along with others, take their medications, and pursue constructive activities. A case manager can coordinate their services and follow them throughout their prison term. With this kind of supportive psychiatric rehab program, many prisoners who might otherwise become victims or chronic inhabitants of security lock-up units are able to create a more productive and stable life for themselves inside prison, and consequently their prognosis and postrelease chances of coping in the community are greatly improved.

Obviously, psychiatric rehabilitation shares much in common with the programs that are lumped under the general rubric of prison rehabilitation. General prison rehabilitation programs, including education, drug counseling, and vocational training opportunities, should be provided for all motivated prisoners, whereas psychiatric rehabilitation is reserved for people who have psychiatric disabilities. But the two forms of rehabilitation programs share many principles. For instance, both aim to increase clients' skills and help them attain the highest quality of life and productivity they are capable of reaching. And both utilize counseling and training to help clients overcome their weaknesses and disabilities.

Psychiatric rehabilitation programs achieve their best results in correctional facilities that also offer a rich variety of general rehabilitation programs. The reason is obvious. In the community, psychiatric rehabilitation programs make use of resources that already exist, including community college programs, factories that are willing to hire psychiatrically disabled workers, low-rent apartments, agencies that accept psychiatrically disabled volunteers, and so forth. The greater the number of these kinds of programs that exist, the more opportunities case managers and staff at halfway houses have to assign their clients to meaningful activities. Likewise, in prisons that contain college classrooms and industrial shops, mental health staff can arrange to have the prisoners they treat assigned to a class or a training slot, and then they can supervise their activities and help them succeed at their assignment in the larger prison rehab program.

## 5. Mental Health Programs for Disturbed Disruptive Prisoners

There is a huge problem managing and treating felons who are considered both "mad" and "bad." I prefer Hans Toch's term for these felons: "disturbed disruptive." Most prison systems lack adequate treatment settings and programs for these prisoners. For instance, in most state prisons inmates are refused admittance to a psychiatric inpatient unit if they have a record of repeated violent episodes. They tend to wind up in supermaximum security housing units, where the harsh conditions and forced idleness worsen their mental disorders, followed by more disruptive behaviors on their part and even longer terms in lock-up.

This group of prisoners present a difficult challenge to correctional as well as mental health staff. The majority of them will serve their terms and be released some day. But if they are merely left in their cells for the remainder of their fixed terms, they are very likely to get into serious trouble immediately after they are released. As I mention in Chapter Three, this group of "mad" and "bad" felons needs a specially designed program that can provide the security necessary to prevent violence as well as the treatment necessary to minimize isolation and regression. They need a way back into the social milieu, facilitated and supervised by experts on violent offenders.

This kind of attention and planning requires resources. A disturbed disruptive inmate requires more staffing, not less, than his easier-to-manage counterpart. This is probably why so many of these prisoners are warehoused in cells and merely given psychiatric medications. But the short-term savings in staff time are a false economy, since this kind of warehousing merely makes these prisoners more rageful and their psychiatric condition deteriorates further. They become a greater long-term management problem and therefore an even greater drain on prison resources, and eventually a greater threat to public safety.

Toch advocates the use of "social learning theory" with the disturbed disruptive prisoner, beginning with an analysis of the prisoner's pattern of misbehavior. Why does a prisoner or a group of prisoners act disruptively when they do? Is there a structural problem on the unit such as unsanitary meals? Is there an especially abusive officer on a particular shift who sets them off? Do the disruptions occur after the prisoners are denied time on the yard? Does the prisoner need psychiatric medications? Has he recently learned that his wife is having an affair, planning to divorce him and take their children? By deploying more staff, the patterns can be uncovered and treatment strategies can be devised.

## 6. Peer Review and Quality Assurance

It is not possible to draw up a standard set of guidelines that will guarantee the quality and adequacy of mental health services in all correctional settings. Accreditation is a useful reminder that there *are* standards, but the standards are only as solid as the good faith of those who are required to reach them. One way to increase the likelihood that an institution will sincerely attempt to reach the accepted standards is to run an honest and efficient peer review and quality assurance program.

Peer review requires meetings of peers to monitor the quality of professional work. Physicians on hospital staffs meet regularly as a committee to evaluate the work of each physician on the staff. Questions about the professional performance of a physician, for instance those raised by a preventable death, are reviewed by a committee of peers. An errant physician might receive a rebuke from the committee, a suspended sentence, a requirement of proctoring by another physician, or a recommendation that the physician not be granted renewal of his staff privileges.

Generally, peer review committees limit their deliberations to the quality of each physician's practice. When the performance and adequacy of an entire program is being considered, another kind of self-examination has to take place. For example, suppose there is an outbreak of staph infections on a hospital ward. Several patients have died from it. The hospital administration calls a meeting of doctors, nurses, and other ward personnel and the whole group makes plans to control the epidemic and prevent future occurrences. While the purpose of this meeting is quality assurance, a purpose shared with peer review, the focus of this meeting is the outbreak, not necessarily the question of a specific professional's ethics or competence. And the meeting is not limited to one professional group.

All concrete plans for the adequate provision of mental health services involve approximations. How many psychiatric inpatient beds are needed in a prison that contains 5,000 convicts? There is no absolute number. Many factors must be considered. For instance, the number of hospital beds that are required depends on the kinds of services that are available to prisoners outside the psychiatric wards. In a prison with sufficient staff to permit adequate attention to all prisoners in need, relatively few hospital beds might be needed. Where the hospital is not the only place a prisoner can talk to a professional therapist, many prisoners will receive help with their emotional problems before they reach the bursting point and have to be hospitalized.

When asked by a judge about possible remedies for the inadequacies of a prison mental health delivery system, I recommend including a first-rate peer review and quality assurance procedure and delegating to these committees tasks such as determining the number of hospital beds needed in their setting. But I quickly add this qualification: a quality assurance committee is only as adequate as its sincerity and commitment to ensure quality care. It is very easy for an institution that falls far short of the minimum standards to set up a peer review and quality assurance committee that merely rubber stamps the current program. An accrediting team reviewing the minutes of the committee's meetings would get the impression that the institution satisfies the standards. The same uncaring attitude that compromises the facility's clinical services can also compromise the staff's will to carry out meaningful quality assurance.

It is important to mention here the private, for-profit corporations that contract to run prisons and their health and mental health services. There is a built-in danger: Private companies tend to maximize their profits by cutting corners and by enlarging the number of people they contract to manage. Where this strategy translates into thinner mental health staffs and services, prisoners with mental disorders suffer undue harm. Where the private contractor is paid on a "capitation basis" to provide mental health services—a flat fee based on the size of the prison population—the company has a financial incentive to diagnose fewer prisoners with mental disorders and to provide less comprehensive treatment. And where the private prison company is paid a certain amount for each prisoner serving time, there is an incentive to cause the prisoners to fail to go straight so they will be returned to prison and serve longer sentences. I wish I were inventing these cynical strategies out of thin air, but unfortunately we have already seen evidence of private companies profiting from their systematic failure to correct. Although it would not be fair to ask peer review and quality assurance committees to take on the entire burden of monitoring private corporations to make sure they do not compromise the quality of clinical services in the interest of maximizing profits, conscientious committees can serve to control some of this kind of abuse.

Ongoing outside monitoring by the courts or by independent watchdog agencies is always a good idea. Where possible, for instance in prisons located near a university medical center, it is also a good idea to have the correctional professional staff and the university medical staff meet jointly for the purposes of peer review and quality assurance.

## 7. Continuity of Care

Aftercare plans and liaison work between prison mental health staff and their counterparts in the community are sorely needed. The majority of prisoners, including those with severe and persistent mental disorders, will eventually serve their full sentence and be released. Some will recycle between community treatment agencies and correctional facilities. It does little good to provide them with excellent care in prison and then set them loose with no treatment or support services on the outside. As part of the treatment plan inside prison, social workers or other outreach liaison workers must remain in touch with the prisoners' families, work with agencies in the community, and do all that is possible to facilitate a smooth transition to postrelease life in the community. A prison treatment program is not really viable if it does not provide comprehensive postrelease services.

## 8. Confidentiality and Access to Care

Confidentiality is a crucial issue. The male code makes it problematic for prisoners to admit they have problems, much less visit "the shrink" to talk about them. This is why a mental health professional who walks up to prisoners' cells and asks them whether they want to talk gets so few positive responses. But if measures are taken to guarantee that prisoners who want to talk can make an entirely confidential appointment to see a clinician and can speak to that clinician in private, a much larger number of prisoners will take advantage of elective mental health services.

For correctional mental health staff to promise prisoners that their conversation will remain confidential is not always possible. There are many instances where the staff member must report what is said to security staff and the administration, for instance when a prisoner discloses something that involves a threat to prison security. But the helping professional can promise the prisoner that she will be straightforward with him about the ground rules regarding confidentiality, and she will follow an ethical code in deciding what to report and to whom. Then the prisoner can decide what can safely be told to the care provider.

The issue of confidentiality comes up often in group therapies. A prisoner who meets with a psychologist in private might expect him to maintain some semblance of confidentiality, but the situation is more complicated for the prisoners in a group therapy. Can a prisoner trust his fellow convicts to guard his secrets? If he admits he is afraid of a tough con, or concerned that his wife might be having an affair, will another member of the group put the word out on the yard? Skilled group leaders have methods for helping prisoners work through complex issues like this, and the working through is, in many cases, a critical part of the treatment. Learning to trust others, and discriminating sufficiently to determine when not to trust them, is a social skill that will come in handy inside as well as outside the walls.

## 9. Separation of Mental Health and Disciplinary Issues

A certain degree of independence from security staff is required if mental health staff are to provide humane treatment. Of course, security is a primary consideration in penal institutions. Mental health staff cannot do their work if the facility is not safe. But too often the routine is so entrenched that security staff call the shots even when a prisoner's actions are not a serious threat to anyone's safety and are clearly the result of her psychiatric condition. Correctional mental health and security staff need to figure out a form of collaboration that does not make treatment considerations entirely subservient to security concerns.

Sometimes clinical staff have to resist the will of security officers. For instance, it is not ethical for a mental health clinician to tell a rape victim that she will not receive treatment unless she first identifies her assailant. When that tactic is employed by correctional officers to foster informing, the mental health clinician has an ethical obligation to object strenuously.

When behaviors on the part of mentally disordered prisoners—including suicide attempts, self-mutilation, rule-breaking, and even some minor violent incidents—are secondary to their mental disorder, they should not be handled entirely as disciplinary infractions requiring punishment. Too often, disruptive acts are merely punished and the possibility that they reflect an imminent psychotic episode or a need for immediate psychiatric attention is never even considered.

This is not to say that staff should excuse impermissible behaviors on the part of mentally disordered prisoners, rather that the behaviors need to be addressed in the context of a treatment plan, a plan that includes careful attention to security issues. The mentally disordered prisoner should not be permitted to accumulate a long term in lock-up. When a posthumous disciplinary write-up for self-destructive acts appears on the chart of a prisoner who has succeeded at suicide, we see how countertherapeutic and perverse the punitive approach can become.

## 10. Cross-Training, Including Cultural Sensitivities

If they are to remain safe *and* supply effective services, mental health staff need to understand the principles that guide the work of correctional officers. And correctional officers need a firm foundation in the principles of psychiatry and mental health treatment if they are to understand and effectively intervene with the large number of prisoners who suffer from mental disorders. The correctional officer is often the first to notice a prisoner's impending emotional breakdown or suicidality. And the mental health clinician is often the one who first realizes that a prisoner who is being punished is actually very disturbed and requires emergency psychiatric treatment. In addition to cross-training, there needs to be close collaboration between the different kinds of staff.

Since prison populations are extraordinarily diverse in terms of race and culture, all staff need to undergo extensive training in diversity issues and cultural sensitivity. I repeatedly hear from prisoners, even when they are not charging overt racism, that the staff are incredibly ignorant of their ethnic background and insensitive to their culture. Although there are many diversity training programs in the community, and they report great success intervening to reduce discrimination in public and private workplaces, none of the prison systems I have toured has made any serious attempt to involve large parts of their staff in this kind of training. It is not possible to provide quality correctional mental health services without giving serious attention to cultural and diversity issues.

---

I regret having to break the news: We need to spend money to establish adequate mental health services behind bars. The relevant principle is that spending some money up-front means spending less in the long run. The imprisonment of a mentally ill person is an illustration of this principle in action. The public mental health system in the community is reeling from massive budget reductions, requiring closure of many outpatient treatment facilities and shorter stays in hospitals and residential halfway houses. But these budget reductions constitute false economizing. If the individual patient was permitted to visit a psychotherapist on a regular basis, spend more time talking to a psychiatrist, or stay in a halfway house long enough to get his bearings, he would be less likely to recycle into the psychiatric inpatient ward or be arrested. And since inpatient services are very expensive, the cost of treating a mental patient who is readmitted to the hospital several times in a year is much greater than the relatively inexpensive provision of halfway house accommodations for the entire year.

A comparison of the costs involved in operating the current correctional system with the cost of effective psychiatric and drug treatment exposes the pure folly of confining seriously mentally ill felons in our harsh, overcrowded prisons. If the mental patient with inadequate treatment runs afoul of the law and is incarcerated, the cost of court proceedings and imprisonment far exceed the cost that would have been entailed in providing sufficient community mental health services to help that individual avoid arrest. The cost of a halfway house in the community is approximately $6,800 per year, the cost of semimonthly supportive outpatient psychotherapy is approximately $2,000 per year, and the cost of methadone maintenance is approximately $3,900 per year. Compare that total with the cost of incarceration, which far exceeds $30,000 per year if any kind of high-security housing or psychiatric care is needed.

Employing the same principle inside our prisons, it would certainly cost something to upgrade prison mental health services, but if adequate treatment prevented a significant number of mentally ill prisoners from being sent to the SHU or being re-arrested after they are released, it would be money very well-spent and would lead to massive savings in the long run.

## Changes in the Entire Prison System

None of the recommendations I've made regarding mental health services will ameliorate the negative mental health effects of idleness and a lack of visitation in the prisons. And no amount of improvement in correctional mental health services will counter the destructive practice of housing mentally ill felons in punitive lockup units. If mentally ill prisoners are to have a better chance of remaining stable and succeeding in their attempts to cope in the community after they are released, large changes are needed in the way our prisons are run. For instance, educational and rehabilitation programs must be bolstered, the quality of visitation must be improved, prisoners' rights must be expanded, and there must be an end to supermaximum security units. It would also serve to improve the mental health of prisoners to break large prisons down into smaller units.

### Bolster Rehabilitation and Educational Programs

I have contrasted psychiatric rehabilitation with general prison rehabilitation and pointed out how the two overlap. Clearly, psychiatric rehabilitation can only be effective with prisoners suffering from serious mental disorders if the prison system encourages and supports all the varieties of rehabilitation. Patients undergoing psychiatric rehabilitation can then make use of the general rehab programs while preparing for postrelease adjustment in the community.

I also have mentioned that the presence of serious educational programs in prison is the factor most strongly correlated with prisoners' chances to succeed at "going straight." Some prisoners take courses from instructors—who are paid to work in the institutions or volunteer their time—while others take courses by mail. Whereas the three-year recidivism rate for all ex-prisoners is between 41 and 63 percent, prisoners who complete their Graduate Equivalency Degree (GED) or a substantial number of college courses while incarcerated have a recidivism rate between 5 and 20 percent. Yet federal Pell grants for prisoners, which enabled prisoners to take college courses, were discontinued by the federal government in 1994. We need to reinstate Pell grants for prisoners and take even stronger actions to maximize the number of prisoners taking part in high school and college classes. Mentally ill prisoners who are able to concentrate and take classes tell me that the opportunity to study and the sense of accomplishment that comes from completing a college course bolster their self-esteem and help them stay out of trouble.

There is heated debate about the efficacy of general prison rehabilitation programs. Detractors say that rehabilitation programs never worked: "These people just don't know the value of an honest job." Its advocates claim that it was never given a chance—there was too little funding in the first place, and with the explosive growth of the prison population since 1980 and the prevailing "get tough" attitude toward convicts, it is political suicide for a governor or legislator to mention upgrading rehab in the prisons.

In 1974 Robert Martinson, a well-respected criminologist, released a comprehensive survey of available outcome studies and concluded that rehabilitation programs have a negligible effect on recidivism rates. Martinson's declaration provided a much-needed rationale for legislators and correctional administrators who were intent on cutting rehabilitation programs. Five years later Martinson withdrew his earlier conclusion that nothing works, and conceded that some prison rehabilitation programs do work, as measured by a reduction in recidivism, if a well-designed program is tailored to specific populations and there is adequate follow-up support after the offender is released. In other words, if we merely correlate the overall recidivism rate with the presence of any kind of rehab program in the prisons, rehabilitation causes no reduction in the overall recidivism rate; but if we look at the outcomes of specific programs for specific subgroups of inmates—for instance, educational programs for motivated prisoners or job training for unskilled youthful offenders—participation in rehab programs has a very positive effect on recidivism rates for these subpopulations.

Of course, some hardcore criminals are uninterested in changing their ways, so their participation in rehabilitation programs has no effect on their recidivism rate. Many other prisoners want very much to "go straight" and they grab every opportunity available to improve their chances. Other researchers have found that with juvenile delinquents, the sooner the problem behavior is treated the better the result, and the more time counselors spend with the juvenile offender the more progress is made. With all offenders, the use of more than one treatment modality works better than reliance on a single modality, and the more programs available to offenders after they are released, the better their postrelease adjustment. Nonetheless, conservative lawmakers ignored the more refined research, and continued to quote from Martinson's earlier paper that supposedly demonstrated the total failure of all rehabilitation efforts.

Another factor that makes assessing the efficacy of rehabilitation programs difficult is a paradox built into the funding process. The public believes, naively, that a successful program will continue in operation, so if a program shuts down, it must not have been successful. But in fact, this is quite untrue for many public and nonprofit programs. I know of several community-based programs that were designed to keep troubled youth from getting into further scrapes with the law by providing mentors, education, and job-training. But when a request was submitted for renewal of funding at the end of three years, it was denied. The executive director of one such program appealed to the federal agency involved, only to be told that the agency recognized the program's success but had to spread its limited resources too thinly to be able to provide funding to any single program beyond a three-year pilot project. Similarly, in prisons, rehabilitation programs that might have been very successful were forced to close, not because of any program failure but merely on account of political trends and funding exigencies.

An even more profound criticism of research on the efficacy of prison rehabilitation is the failure to consider the negative effects of crowding and harsh prison conditions. Just as inner-city children who are traumatized cannot pay attention and learn their lessons in school, prisoners who are massively traumatized cannot participate effectively in rehabilitation programs. The prisoner who has to sleep in a noisy makeshift dorm, the victim of prison rape, the mother upset about a child's situation, the prisoner who is denied quality visits with loved ones, or is suffering from a severe mental disorder—all of these prisoners are unable to make optimal use of rehabilitation programs. Their failures result more from the overwhelming stresses of life in overcrowded and harshly punitive institutions than from any lack of motivation or interest in self-improvement.

Finally, there is the problem of a lack of continuity and follow-through in the programs that do exist. It is one thing to train a prisoner in a trade, but if that prisoner is unable to find work after being released, or is given insufficient postrelease supervision to stay clear of drugs and the old criminal ways, that training will have been wasted and the prisoner will soon wind up back behind bars. A rehabilitation program is viable only if it is linked with comprehensive postrelease services, including aggressive efforts to help the ex-prisoner overcome stigma and find meaningful work.

## Improve Visitation

In Chapter Seven I point out that quality visitation helps a convict avoid trouble while incarcerated and correlates strongly with postrelease success. This is especially true for felons suffering from severe and lasting mental disorders. I also explain some built-in dynamics that make visitation problematic. Those dynamics need to be reexamined so that prisoners and their loved ones can have quality visits.

Prisoners should be assigned to facilities near their homes so their families can visit. Visiting hours should be extended, where appropriate, so that more visitation can occur, especially with children. Far fewer prisoners should be kept in lock-up units and forced to visit through glass while shackled. Prisoners should be permitted to wear their personal clothing during visits. Conjugal or family visiting programs should be expanded to include more prisoners and their families. Furloughs should be granted so that prisoners who pose no escape risk and are cooperating with their prison program can be permitted to go home to visit their families. And prisoners who get into trouble should not be moved far away from their families—contact with people who love them tends to help these prisoners rein in their tempers and tolerate the stress of prison life. In every way feasible, correctional staff should foster the best visiting possible for every prisoner.

## Attend to Prisoners' Rights

The more prisoners feel they are being treated unfairly, the more turmoil and violence occur in the prisons. A warden can be tough and institute strict but fair disciplinary procedures, and the prisoners will accept the toughness relatively well. But if the rules are arbitrary, if the hearing panels almost always rule in favor of security officers, if prisoners of color have to appear before entirely white hearing panels and appeal boards, the prisoners are going to feel they are being denied a fair hearing, they are going to feel they have "nothing to lose," and they are going to have less incentive to follow the rules and avoid violence.

Prison disciplinary procedures need to be reexamined. Where possible, the rules need to be spelled out clearly. Prisoners need recourse when they feel unjustly accused. Hearing panels should be of the same racial and cultural diversity as the population of prisoners, and there should be a significant proportion of nonstaff members, including prisoners and ex-prisoners, on the panels. Prisoners should be able to mount a case in their defense, with outside legal counsel when appropriate, or at least with the help of an ombudsman or prisoner advocate who is not beholden to the warden or biased in favor of the staff. In terms of parole boards, Dr. Lige Dailey recommends that 50 percent of the members should be ex-prisoners—an excellent idea.

We also need to reconsider the tendency in recent years to reduce prisoners' access to the courts. The reduction of access takes many forms, but one example is the clause in the federal Prison Litigation Reform Act that cancels the waiver of filing fees for indigent prisoners. Most prisoners are indigent, so that clause essentially means that even if their case has great merit they will be unable to gain access to the courts. That is just one of many recent changes in the law that diminish prisoners' fair redress of grievances. The overall effect is to increase a sense of hopelessness among prisoners, which decreases their motivation to stay out of trouble. Maximizing prisoners' sense of fairness and just redress would improve relations between prisoners and staff, help maintain the peace, decrease the stress that leads to so many emotional breakdowns and suicides, and help prisoners prepare for and succeed at postrelease adjustment in the community.

## End Long-Term Lock-Up, Including Supermax Security

The housing of an expanding population of prisoners in supermaximum control units is not only failing as a method for reducing violence in the prisons, it is actually increasing the violence and mental disturbance. We know that a significant number of mentally disturbed prisoners find their way into prison lock-up units. These are the mentally ill prisoners who act out their rage instead of turning it inward and hiding in their cells. And we know that time spent in a lock-up facility causes emotional damage and intensified resentment in almost all prisoners, but especially in those who are prone to psychiatric decompensation.

Even where there are court orders to keep mentally disordered felons out of the SHU, as at California's Pelican Bay State Prison, a significant number remain there. In part, this is because correctional authorities tend to interpret the rule-breaking and violence of mentally disordered felons as signs of their "badness," not their "madness." And in part this is because the quality of mental health screening and monitoring is poor, causing the signs of impending psychiatric breakdown to go unnoticed. In any case, the fact that so many mentally disturbed felons wind up in the supermaximum security units around the country is reason enough to close them down. But an additional reason is the tendency for these units to cause emotional damage in prisoners who don't have a history of prior psychiatric problems.

We know from psychological research that punishment only works if it is meted out fairly, tailored to specific behaviors, and is immediate and short-lived enough to foster motivation for positive change. In the old days, when a prisoner was "thrown in the hole" for ten days or a month after getting into a fight or being caught with a shank (a knife made from found objects), the punishment served to eradicate the undesirable behaviors. I do not mean to create nostalgia for the old days—in the hands of sadistic wardens and guards, "the hole" became a place of torture. The point is that all other variables being equal, short-term punishments have the best chance of improving behaviors. But when prisoners are sentenced to lock-up for years at a time, the prisoner loses hope of ever getting out. The rage builds, the prisoner feels he has nothing to lose, and as soon as he believes he is being unfairly "hassled" by a correctional officer or another prisoner he strikes out. When prisoners get out of supermax units, they tend to be so full of rage and so disoriented by their time in isolation that they end up being meaner, more disturbed, more violent, and more likely to break the law than they were before they were sent to the SHU.

After closing down the supermaximum security units, we will have to devise a better way to handle the prisoners who repeatedly get into fights and create disturbances. We will also have to figure out a method to cope with gangs. All this would not be nearly as difficult if there were less crowding, more rehabilitation programs, better quality visitation, and fairer disciplinary procedures. With all of these changes in place, it would be possible, in every case where a prisoner repeatedly gets into trouble, for staff to embark on a thorough evaluation of his gripes and an energetic individualized plan to manage him more effectively. Then there would be no need for long-term lock-up.

## Create Smaller Facilities

Large correctional facilities containing thousands of prisoners tend to be administrative nightmares. Staff move about from one cellblock to another, never really getting to know a particular group of prisoners. And prisoners are moved from one setting to another so they never really form trusting bonds with anyone. The warden is unable to get to know his correctional officers, much less all of the prisoners under his control.

Imagine for a minute what would happen if the prisons were broken down into units with a maximum occupancy of 500 prisoners, and each smaller facility had a warden or superintendent of its own and a group of staff, including mental health practitioners, who worked only in that institution. In addition, imagine that all prisoners would remain in that facility for their entire time behind bars. There would be administrative segregation units and other forms of "lock-up," but no prisoner would be permanently housed in them. The staff and prisoners would get to know each other, and all problems would have to be dealt with on the premises.

Of course, where there are sadistic staff and an indifferent warden, the size of the facility cannot guarantee a humane program. But where there is a competent warden who is committed to rehabilitating felons, or at least providing them with a decent environment to do their time, a creative staff would have opportunities to solve problems together in a more manageable facility. The correctional staff and mental health staff could meet together to brainstorm about how to manage the mentally disturbed prisoner, the rowdy prisoner, the rapist, and the potential rape victim. Everyone would get to know everyone else and there would be an incentive for everyone to get along and try to solve all problems that emerge.

## Changes in the Entire Criminal Justice System

We need a bold wish list if we really want to envision a more effective and humane system of criminal justice. Obviously, we need to address the social problems that make crime and violence endemic in our society. As a society, we need to attend to the pathetic condition of public education in our inner cities, the lack of meaningful employment prospects for disadvantaged youth, the problem of poverty, the urgent need for adequate low-cost housing, and restoration of the safety net that used to be provided by social welfare programs. We need to end the pervasive racism that perpetuates the disproportionate imprisonment of people of color. And we need to bolster and upgrade the public mental health system.

The National Criminal Justice Commission has proposed a thoughtful list of corrections to the massive problems and inequities that plague our criminal justice system, including

- Calling for a three-year moratorium on new prison construction
- Approaching substance abuse as a public health problem rather than a criminal matter
- Eliminating racial and ethnic biases in criminal justice
- Reducing violence by employing public health strategies and passing serious gun control legislation
- Reducing poverty by investing in children, youth, families, and communities

John Irwin and James Austin also recommend reducing the prison population by shortening sentences across the board.

Jerome Miller recommends

Halting the "war on drugs" and the associated "sting operations" and reliance on "snitches" to gather information

Diverting as many young offenders as possible out of the criminal justice system

Establishing meaningful affirmative action policies for the staff of criminal justice agencies

Bolstering educational, employment, and social welfare programs

Persevering, not giving up, on entire groups of young offenders we deem "incorrigible"

I heartily endorse the recommendations proposed by the Commission, John Irwin and James Austin, and Jerome Miller, and I believe the changes they recommend would have a very positive effect on the plight of mentally disordered offenders and felons.

I will comment about a few key items: Creating alternatives to incarceration for mentally ill offenders as well as substance abusers who have not been convicted of violent crimes, putting an end to racial disparities in the criminal justice system as well as overcrowding in the prisons, and directing a significant proportion of our resources toward interventions with young offenders.

## Create Alternatives for Offenders with Mental Disorders

There are two parts to this recommendation. We need to address the shifts in social welfare policy and law that have led in recent years to widespread arrests and incarceration of people suffering from serious and persistent mental disorders, and we need to provide alternative punishments for mentally disturbed people who do break the law.

In Chapter Two I outline some of the shifts in social welfare policy and law that have led to the imprisonment of a large number of mentally ill felons. The promise of deinstitutionalization was to establish community mental health centers capable of providing adequate services to mental patients who would no longer reside in state hospitals. But the budget for public mental health services has been progressively reduced ever since. A large number of mentally ill citizens are left adrift in the community, their safety net destroyed as social welfare programs are cut, and a certain number get into trouble.

Here's where the shifts in the law come in. There is less sympathy today for lawbreakers, especially violent offenders, so a growing proportion of disturbed people who get into trouble go to jail or prison. If we are to improve the plight of the mentally ill in our jails and prisons, we have greatly to improve the public mental health system, reverse the cuts in social welfare of the last couple of decades, and rethink the legal issues involved in sending mentally disturbed law breakers into brutal prisons. Essentially, this society has been deinstitutionalizing the mentally ill out of psychiatric facilities and then reinstitutionalizing a large proportion in jails and prisons.

Some mental health practitioners are arguing we should reopen the state mental hospitals so that this population can stay out of trouble. Others propose better systems of public mental health care in the community. In either case, we need to reconsider our social priorities and recognize that cutting the budget for public mental health services merely forces an expansion of the corrections budget, and leads to a great amount of suffering and disability for people with serious mental disorders who land in prison.

## Divert Drug Offenders and Nonviolent Felons

Not all people convicted of a crime need to go to prison. Someone who is using drugs illegally, but has not been caught robbing to get them or selling them in large amounts, does not need to go to prison. In fact, comparing drug addicts who go to prison and do not take part in a drug treatment program with an equivalent group of addicts who graduate from a well-run drug treatment program in the community, a much greater proportion of the ex-prisoners use drugs a year after they are released.

The explosive growth of the prison population in the last two decades is largely due to the imprisonment of drug offenders, most of whom have never been convicted of a violent crime. Imprisonment does not cut down on their drug use. But when they do not take part in any meaningful rehabilitative services and they are brutalized by guards and fellow prisoners alike, their chances of remaining drug-free and becoming productive citizens after release are greatly diminished. Community alternatives to incarceration for drug offenders are very effective today, and should be ordered by the courts and made available to drug offenders.

## End Racial Disparities in the Entire Criminal Justice System

This is a tall order. Putting an end to racial disparities in arrests, convictions, and laws governing drug crimes and sentencing is absolutely essential if there is to be any real improvement in the plight of mentally ill prisoners. Of course, the only way to do this is to make sweeping changes in social policy and the law, which in turn require a readjustment of social priorities. For instance, we need to make serious attempts to correct the inadequacies of inner-city schools and the dismal lifetime employment prospects faced by young, inner-city youth today. All of this is beyond the scope of this book. But just imagine, in terms of the mental health of prisoners of color, how much less cause there would be for depression, paranoia, and the wish to escape reality, were there real racial equality in the eyes of the law.

## End Crowding Behind Bars

The prison population has quadrupled since 1980, and we know that crowding is correlated with increased prevalences of violence, suicide, and psychiatric decompensation. During the same years there have been a heightened "war on drugs," a dismantling of rehabilitation programs behind bars, and an influx of mentally disordered felons into the prisons. And the increase in prison violence has been used to rationalize incarcerating a growing number of prisoners for long periods in supermaximum security units. Obviously, an end to the crowding would have a ripple effect on other problems.

I have already made recommendations that would help reduce the crowding. If a significant proportion of mentally disordered offenders were diverted to treatment facilities, the prison population would be reduced, as would the degree of psychiatric disability. If nonviolent drug offenders were diverted to drug programs in the community, the prison population would shrink to an even greater extent.

In addition, between 15 and 20 percent of prisoners are in prison at this time because they violated the conditions of their parole. In many cases, the parole violation involved very minor infractions. For instance, many parole departments require unannounced urine tests for drugs and alcohol, and when a parolee's test turns up positive his parole is violated and he is returned to prison. Since we know that time in prison does not help people stay clean and sober, this is an irrational and counterproductive policy. Why not divert parolees who turn in positive urine tests to mandatory drug treatment programs in the community? This would also reduce the prison population.

There are many other ways to reduce the size of the prison population. We need to reexamine all our laws and sentencing guidelines and create a more rational, fair, and humane criminal justice system. The crime rate in most categories has been relatively flat for the last quarter of a century. No one knows whether the decrease of a few points in the last few years is a result of changes in criminal justice policies or merely a reflection of population demographics. For example, there are fewer males between the ages of sixteen and twenty-five today, and that is the age group responsible for a preponderance of crime. But in spite of a relatively flat crime rate, the imprisonment rate has been steadily growing.

Although there are a certain number of hard-core criminals who must be quarantined for the protection of society, it is not possible that there could be four times as many of these people today as there were in 1980. Rather, it is clear that imprisonment rates are more related to social priorities than they are to crime rates, and in the last two decades our social policies have aimed at "disappearing" large segments of the population, including extremely disproportionate numbers of poor people and people of color. We need to reexamine our social priorities and our sentencing guidelines. And we need to reduce drastically the number of people we send to prison.

## Concentrate Resources on Rehabilitating Young Offenders

Everyone I know who works with young offenders reports that their programs and interventions are effective. I have not focused on young offenders in this book, but I add this recommendation here because it is so obvious and crucial if we really want to make the criminal justice system more just and effective. When adequate funding permits serious counselors and community organizers to intervene to reduce gang violence, drug use, and crime among young people, the results are impressive. Alternatively, when young offenders are sent to correctional institutions many of them are traumatized and learn that their options are limited to a life of crime and violence.

Consider a hypothetical life history of a mentally disordered adult felon. He was probably abused and abandoned as a child; he probably failed in school and drifted into crime and drugs instead of finding meaningful employment. With the added stress of unemployment, illicit drugs, a lack of family support, and trouble with the law, he experienced his first psychotic episode in his late teens or early twenties. Whether his first breakdown occurred in a correctional setting or in the community, after he developed a severe and persistent mental illness he became increasingly dysfunctional and eventually was convicted of a crime and received a long prison sentence.

If we think for a moment about when we could have intervened most effectively to help this individual avoid a life of crime and imprisonment, it's obvious that the earlier we could have done so the better would have been our chances of helping him. If, when he came to the attention of a court as a teenager, he had been diverted into a community program where his learning deficits could have been corrected and he could have been trained in a line of work, he might have been able to enter the workforce and establish a constructive life for himself in the community. He might still have suffered an emotional breakdown, but his condition probably would have been recognized more quickly and psychiatric care could have been provided to help him restabilize his life and return to work. Alternatively, if he was sent to prison during his late adolescence, his psychiatric disability would certainly have resulted in his being victimized or thrown into a lock-up unit, and psychiatric treatment would have been inadequate. The point of this hypothetical exercise is that early attention to the problems of a youthful offender, diversion into a noncorrectional program, and rapid initiation of mental health services, where they are indicated, would greatly increase the likelihood of his eventually becoming a productive and law-abiding citizen.

---

I have outlined some changes in social policies and priorities that would greatly improve the situation in our prisons as well as the plight of mentally disordered convicts. Many other recommendations could be added to the list. The point is we need to begin to initiate changes at all three levels. The tragic situation in our prisons requires urgent action.

## Some Model Programs

I know of no ideal prison system. Most American prisons are overcrowded, provide few opportunities for rehabilitation, offer very inadequate mental health services, and contain psychosis-inducing supermaximum control units. Still, within these very flawed systems there are some valiant attempts to create humane, innovative, and effective programs. Even if these attempts eventually fail, it is worth studying the experience gained with subpopulations of felons so that we can identify the kinds of programs that are effective in rehabilitating felons and we can plan for the day when more rational criminal justice policies will permit departments of corrections to make use of the models to create better prison systems. A look outside the United States for effective models is also useful.

### Model Programs in American Prisons

There are exceptions to the cruel policies that prevail in American prisons today, and some model programs display a remarkable level of sensitivity to the needs of prisoners. But most of the model programs are too small to reach the majority of prisoners. In many cases, these model programs are terminated just when they begin to have a positive impact, often for very unclear reasons. Meanwhile, the prisons are currently being inundated with a huge number of new admissions and the resulting overcrowding inhibits all efforts to rehabilitate prisoners.

Each prison system has its pet projects and model programs. Usually admission to these programs is very restrictive. For instance, as I mention in Chapter Five, California's state prison system for women contains a residential program in the community where pregnant felons can be housed until they give birth and have an opportunity to get to know their newborn child. But only low-security women felons can gain access to that residential program, and the spaces are very limited. In fact, most pregnant prisoners are unaffected by the existence of the program. Although it is admirable that the California prison system has instituted a program that permits a few pregnant prisoners to bear their children outside the prison walls, it is cruel to deny that opportunity to a large proportion of the pregnant women inside.

Prisoner/author Kathy Boudin has created a program for mothers at Bedford Hills state prison in New York called "Parenting from a Distance." Boudin leads groups for prisoners who are mothers, modeled on women's consciousness-raising groups that evolved in the late 1960s, where women talk about their sense of powerlessness, their shame, and their guilt about not being available to their children. They tell their stories of abuse and disempowerment. They empower themselves by listening to each other's stories and accepting each other in spite of what each of them might have suffered and done in the past. And they talk about their feelings as mothers and how they can be better parents, even from inside prison walls.

Another example of a model program was the Santa Cruz Women's Prison Project conducted by Karlene Faith and other volunteers at the California Institution for Women (CIW) in the 1970s. They discovered that women prisoners were much more intelligent than many of their keepers had assumed. The women's average IQ score on the Stanford-Binet test was 110, well above average for the entire citizenry. They taught courses and found that the women participated with enthusiasm, and the learning process helped them do their time and stay out of trouble. The teachers also reported that they learned a lot from working with women prisoners.

Faith's outcome research showed that only 5 percent of the prisoners who completed credit courses had returned to prison five years after their release, whereas approximately 70 percent of women who did not participate would return to prison in that interval. As often happens, the program was eventually shut down by correctional authorities. The California Department of Corrections bowed to pressure from guards who claimed the program undermined their authority, and they expelled the Santa Cruz Women's Prison Project from CIW.

The Washington State Department of Corrections and the University of Washington are collaborating in the establishment of model programs for the management and treatment of prisoners suffering from serious mental illnesses. For instance, they have set up a treatment center for moderately acute inmates at McNeil Island where community psychiatrists work with correctional staff to design therapeutic programs that meet security needs.

Another collaborative effort by Washington's Department of Corrections and the University of Washington is the Mobile Assessment Program, involving a team of four staff members from other institutions who travel to a prison where a mentally disturbed prisoner is creating a ruckus. The team makes a visit and assesses the situation. Then, from the perspective of outsiders who do not have a history of managing the particular disruptive prisoner, they recommend a management plan, including advice about placing the prisoner in a mental health treatment setting or a punitive detention unit. The visit by a mobile team formed of staff from other institutions provides some objectivity in situations in which a prisoner has earned the animosity of the local staff and staff are feeling less than kind. One hopes the knowledge that a mobile visiting team can be called will help the local staff avoid burnout and despair.

Some of the most promising model programs are in the realm of community alternatives to incarceration and postrelease programs, especially ones designed for young offenders. The best of these programs involve collaboration between mental health providers in the community and correctional mental health staff, multidisciplinary teams that provide a wide range of services, liaisons with job-training agencies and educational institutions in the community, and support from law enforcement agencies and the courts for efforts to divert nonviolent criminals suffering from mental illnesses into noncorrectional treatment settings.

There are many impressive model programs. One hopes that someday an entire prison system will utilize their accumulated wisdom in establishing a better approach to corrections.

## Worldwide Models

We have to keep in mind that each country has its own unique approach to criminology and criminal justice. Crime rates and sentencing practices vary, and so do public attitudes about the social purposes of imprisonment. Still, by examining programs and correctional policies that seem to work well, we can envision worthy improvements for the United States.

Denmark's approach to imprisonment seems very enlightened. The Danes view prisons as just another branch of social services for citizens who have gone astray. They view crime in the context of education, employment, and socioeconomic opportunity. Though they do not believe that prisons are effective in rehabilitating criminals, they are firmly committed to providing a safe, humane environment for people who are sentenced to serve time as punishment for their crimes.

Sentences in Denmark tend to be much shorter than they are in the United States. For example, felons convicted of burglary and larceny serve an average of four to six months in prison, while the comparable averages in the United States are forty-four months for burglary and thirty-seven months for larceny. Unlike Americans, the Danes do not believe that harsh prison conditions serve as a deterrent to crime, and they are optimistic that the majority of criminals will straighten out their own lives if they are given a second chance.

Danish prisons are quite unlike ours. They are much smaller. Whereas prisons in the United States often contain several thousand prisoners, Danish prisons are limited in size to approximately 200. The smaller size, they believe, enables the prisoners and staff to get to know each other and figure out constructive ways to settle their differences. Indeed, there is very little violence between correctional staff and prisoners in Denmark.

One of the most intriguing aspects of correctional philosophy in Denmark is the notion of one prisoner to a cell. The Danes believe that a prisoner needs privacy and a place to escape from the often frenetic prison milieu if he is to reevaluate his life and reform himself. Prisoners are also permitted to decorate their cells, which means that the prisons are not as drab as many in the United States.

Besides being responsible for prison security, the correctional staff serve as vocational instructors, teachers, and social workers. They are responsible for supervising the prisoners as well as training them in the skills they were lacking when they committed their crimes. The prisoners are expected to work or attend school. Idleness is not permitted.

Another feature of Danish prisons is the support that staff provide for continuing family and community ties. Wherever possible, prisoners are housed in institutions near their homes. Family visits are encouraged. Furloughs are permitted as a reward for good behavior. And the Danes are experimenting with "Open Prisons" wherein low-security prisoners are sent into the community to work during the day, returning to the prison to sleep at night.

Other countries have model programs, even where the entire prison system is not as enlightened as Denmark's. For instance, within the Mexican prison system, which contains some rather harsh high-security institutions, is the Tres Marias penal colony for federal convicts serving very long terms. Families can join the prisoners on one of the three islands within the facility, and prisoners are provided with very humane vocational and recreational opportunities. They are able to sustain their social skills and family connections while preparing for their eventual release.

The Netherlands has one of the lowest incarceration rates of any advanced industrial nation. They are committed to the prevention of crowding in their prisons. Like the Danes, they insist on the "one prisoner, one cell" rule because they believe prisoners, like other citizens, are entitled to privacy and respite.

These are a few ideas from other countries. None of the countries I mentioned has a perfect record. It is not even very relevant to compare recidivism rates, since the overall crime rates vary so widely from country to country. But it is always useful to borrow ideas that work. Just imagine prisoners being given their own cells in smaller, uncrowded prisons, having quality visits with loved ones who live nearby, taking part in vocational training and educational programs, and receiving counseling from guards whom they grow to trust. Quite a contrast to what occurs in the United States. How many fewer emotional breakdowns would occur behind bars if this vision is put into practice? And how many more ex-prisoners might eventually go straight?

---

Correctional mental health treatment and rehabilitation programs will only work when the policymakers, correctional staff, and public want them to work. If society wants to treat and rehabilitate its prisoners, if its lawmakers can stand up to the very loud and powerful faction calling for harsher sentences and question the wisdom of throwing money at prisons and the police, and if the public mood grows more generous, there could be a whole new era in corrections. In the final chapter I discuss the flawed logic of law and order that holds us back and I suggest the kind of vision we will need to move forward.

# 11

# The Folly of Law and Order

One big reason for the public's unwillingness to give felons a fair opportunity to rehabilitate themselves or to provide adequate treatment for mentally disordered prisoners is the prevailing logic of law and order. That logic has very deleterious effects on mentally ill felons. A court system intent on harsh punishment is unlikely to take the mental state of a criminal into consideration in the process of deciding on guilt and establishing a sentence. And when an enlarged pool of mentally disordered prisoners arrive in prison and suffer from the harsh conditions, their complaints of cruelty and inadequate treatment meet with little sympathy.

If we are to reform our prisons, and if the mentally ill are to receive adequate care, we need to understand why so many people accept the very flawed logic that guides the imprisonment binge, we need to reject the plan to quarantine a growing population of citizens in brutal institutions, and we need to create a better approach to the problems of crime and mental disability.

## The Flawed Logic of Law and Order

The logic of law and order maintains that a certain number of "bad apples" are responsible for crime and violence, and if they could just be identified and locked up for a very long time the streets would be safe for law-abiding citizens. Advocates of tougher law enforcement, harsher sentences, and "three-strikes-and-you're-out" legislation would also like to cut out rehabilitation programs, weight lifting on prison yards, group therapy, prisoners' access to the courts, and all other forms of "coddling." A society that ascribes to this logic cannot permit itself to be too concerned about the plight of those mentally ill prisoners who are locked up and hidden from the public's view.

But there are serious flaws in this logic. For example, there's a big question about whether it's actually possible to identify, much less round up, a "criminal element." A large proportion of violent crimes are committed by young men who have never served time in prison and who do not seem to be deterred from acts of violence by the prospect of harsher sentences. In addition, not all crimes and not all arrests lead to conviction, so a great many perpetrators remain at large, no matter how draconian the criminal justice system.

The biggest problem with the logic of law and order is this very foolish and dangerous conviction: Since the harshness of prison life and the lack of preparation for going straight make the "bad apples" all the angrier and more prone to criminal activities after they are released, they are more dangerous to society than ever so we should never let them out of prison.

## Disappearing People

Sociologists talk about a line that divides the "deserving" from the "undeserving poor." We believe that physically disabled people deserve disability benefits and medical care because, presumably, their misfortune is not their own fault. But we view criminals as undeserving of public benefits. They chose to do the crime and they have to suffer the consequences, no matter how severe and inhumane.

It seems that mentally ill prisoners have been moved to the "undeserving" side of that line as well. When a person suffering from a serious mental illness is convicted of a crime and sent to prison, his disability benefits are terminated, he is "disappeared" into a brutal world where he is unlikely to receive adequate treatment, and his suffering is quickly forgotten. When the public turns its back on those they put behind prison walls, conditions "inside" deteriorate very rapidly, especially for mentally ill prisoners.

Attitudes toward disenfranchized people seem to vary with the economic situation. In this time of economic uncertainty for all but the most affluent, there is widespread insecurity and a pervasive attitude of taking care of one's own and forgetting about others who cannot take care of themselves—including the homeless, immigrants, teen welfare mothers, the disabled, and especially the criminals. We are at the nadir of sympathy for the "have-nots."

For example, consider our attitude toward homelessness. Instead of demanding more affordable housing so that no one needs to go homeless, there are calls for more laws and ordinances aimed against the homeless, as though there is a wish to expel them from town. Remember when homelessness itself was not a crime, until the homeless made themselves too visible by panhandling at ATM's? Only when they made affluent people uncomfortable were they locked up. Currently, cities are racing to outdo each other, passing ordinances to outlaw sitting or sleeping on public streets, camping in city parks, or panhandling alongside freeway exits. The criminalization of homelessness—one of the ways this society gets rid of the poor as well as a certain number of people with psychiatric disabilities—removes the daily reminders of the obvious injustice of the very existence of homelessness in the richest country in the world. Meanwhile, the prison population expands.

As a general rule, the higher one is situated on the socioeconomic ladder the more public concern there is about one's pain. A human interest story about a movie star or CEO who is struggling with cancer enjoys a larger audience than, for instance, the recent report of research finding that only a small proportion of people who are removed from the welfare roles succeed in finding work. There is shockingly little public concern about the rising number of homeless people who are contracting pneumonia and tuberculosis and dying in our cities.

Like the suffering of poor people in the community, the repetitive traumas in prisoners' lives enjoy very little public attention. Although therapists rush to volunteer their services to survivors of a natural disaster or a school shooting in order to prevent a subsequent outbreak of PTSD, very few volunteer to enter the prisons to work with men and women who have been repeatedly brutalized since childhood. In fact, very few mental health professionals are interested in working in correctional settings, probably because they know that security concerns often make clinical interventions problematic. Underfunded and overstretched prison mental health services aren't able to provide "debriefing" for prisoners who've been brutalized by guards or raped, and very few prisoners are provided an opportunity to sit and talk to a psychotherapist about the physical and sexual abuse they suffered as children or the domestic violence that plagued them as adults.

## Fear and Revenge

Why do voters continue to support politicians who call for harsher prison sentences and divert a growing segment of public resources to building and running prisons at the expense of all other social programs? This is not only a matter of logic. If the prison industry is to grow, the public must be convinced on a gut level that locking up the "bad seed" will solve our social ailments. According to the polls, crime and violence are the social ailments that provoke the most public concern. Health care, housing, and the plight of low-income people are much lower on voters' priority list.

Newspaper headlines and blockbuster movies focus on violent crime while television specials on murder and mayhem lure viewers into phoning in clues to the whereabouts of high-profile killers. As the media play to the public's darkest fears, their depiction of crime and violence enlarge those fears out of proportion to the actual danger that lurks on the streets—remember, crime rates are flat or down by a few points—and of course this enlargement serves to swell their audiences. Meanwhile, a public stirred to irrational fear of criminals is not very likely to complain when public funds are diverted into corrections and prisoners are brutalized.

But fear is not the whole story behind society's allegiance to the logic of law and order. Another theme that appears regularly in the media is a craving for revenge on the part of crime victims and their families. Psychiatrist Karl Menninger, in his seminal work on punishment and rehabilitation, offered this comment about the public's attitude: "The great secret, the deeply buried mystery of the apparent public apathy to crime and to proposals for better controlling crime, lies in the persistent, intrusive wish for vengeance."

A friend told me recently about being robbed on the street at gunpoint. Her assailant threatened to rape her if she did not turn over her purse and jewelry fast enough, and for many nights she had nightmares about being raped and murdered. Our conversation turned to sharing fantasies of capturing the perpetrator, beating him to within an inch of his life, and then turning him over to the police so he could be sent to prison and learn what it feels like to be raped.

Revenge fantasies are understandable on a personal level. They provide an opportunity to vent and regain a lost sense of potency. But as social policy, the revenge motive is very destructive. Genocide, for instance, is always rationalized as revenge for past atrocities committed by the current victims or their forebears. Inhumane prisons may seem to provide greater safety on the streets and revenge for the victims of violent crime, but it is becoming very clear that harsh treatment and lack of rehabilitative opportunities actually increase the likelihood that released felons will act out their growing rage in further violent acts.

Revenge does not make for good social policy. A citizenry that identifies criminals as the singular source of their fears and makes revenge a central part of its social policy soon discovers that this kind of diffuse resentment and distrust can be shifted to other groups at any time. When vengeance dominates our public sensibility, selfishness and distrust grow while the spirit of community wanes.

## Creating a Greater Problem

There is a big flaw in the logic of law and order: When awful things are done to prisoners and their emotional needs are ignored, they become more resentful and more likely to repeat the kinds of illegal acts that landed them in prison. Some will become more prone to violence. Felons who were already mentally disturbed when they entered prison will become more disturbed. Another group who were emotionally stable prior to incarceration will go mad.

Whereas it is important to clarify that mentally disordered prisoners as a group are no more violence-prone than nondisturbed prisoners, a subgroup of prisoners who have difficulty controlling their tempers and spend most of their prison terms in solitary confinement do pose a very serious threat to public safety. When the prisons are overcrowded, prisoners are relatively idle and a significant proportion do their time in lock-up units; a certain number of ex-prisoners—but not the majority—commit horrendous crimes soon after they are released. Is it really wise to put prisoners who have not been convicted of a violent crime, mentally ill people, and violent felons together in overcrowded and brutal institutions?

When I was in Michigan to testify in *Cain* v. *MDOC*, Matt Davis, a spokesperson for the MDOC, responded on television news to my concern that the proposed policy depriving prisoners of most of their possessions would have detrimental effects on their mental health: "They should have thought about that before they robbed, raped, and killed people. I mean, that's what these prisoners have done. These aren't prisoners who have a human identity. They are prisoners, they have committed sins, cardinal sins, original sins, against Michigan's citizens."

Of course, as a representative of a large state department of corrections, Mr. Davis must be aware of the fact that a huge majority of prisoners have never "raped and killed" anyone, and he must also know that treating people as if they have no "human identity" only results in their becoming even more rageful and less likely to abide by the law. The logic of law and order calls for exaggeration and distortion at every turn.

Advocates of law and order have an answer to concerns about brutalized prisoners being released: "But that's precisely our point, felons are evil people and most of them need to be locked up and never released." In other words, whether or not crowded prisons that lack rehabilitation and psychiatric treatment programs and resort to supermaximum security detention cause prisoners to be more dangerous, the solution is even more time in prison under even harsher conditions.

This response, like Mr. Davis's suggestion that we relate to prisoners as though they have no "human identity," is a recipe for disaster. Here is the madness in this society's current approach to corrections. Either we will need to keep a huge number of prisoners behind bars for the remainder of their lives, or we are designing correctional institutions that will actually create more of a threat to public safety.

I have to admit that as progressive prison reformers we weaken our argument whenever we appear to ignore the public's intense fears about crime, or when we try to minimize the fact that there really are some people who do terrible things and deserve to be in prison for a very long time. There needs to be more sensitivity toward the public's very real concerns. To say that prisoners should not be brutalized, or that those with mental disorders should receive adequate treatment, is not to say they should get off scot-free. But to say that the things we do to prisoners makes them more desperate and more of a threat to public safety is not to say that they should be locked away forever.

## The Hidden Agenda Behind Our Imprisonment Binge

Anyone who takes the trouble to garner the facts, avoids the subjective distortions arising from fear and a need for vengeance, and seriously analyzes the way our prisons are run will come to the conclusion that our prisons are designed to fail. Of course, success and failure have to be measured in relation to the aims of institutions. Perhaps the transparency of the failure that is built into the design provides a clue about why our correctional system is so bad at "correcting" the people who are sent to prison. Inevitably, an exploration of this issue leads to our questioning who profits from the failure. Those who have seen through the false logic of law and order eventually arrive at the much more rational notion of a Prison-Industrial Complex that fosters the false logic in the interest of maximizing profits and power.

### Designed to Fail?

We know that prison overcrowding causes increased rates of violence, psychiatric breakdown, and suicide, yet we keep pouring more people into our prisons. We know that well-designed rehabilitation programs help prisoners prepare for "going straight" whereas idleness leads to violence and emotional disability, yet we keep on dismantling prison rehabilitation programs. We know that prisoners who take part in college classes have a markedly reduced recidivism rate, yet we bar prisoners from utilizing federal Pell grants to take college courses. We know that rapid and effective psychiatric intervention with acute psychiatric breakdowns leads to better outcomes and prognoses, yet our correctional mental health services are so inadequate that many psychotic prisoners have to wait a long time to be diagnosed and even longer to be transferred to an acute inpatient facility. We know that quality visitation correlates strongly with successful postrelease adjustment, yet we situate high-security prisons far from population centers and create endless bureaucratic roadblocks to family visits.

We know that solitary confinement in lock-up units causes severe mental health problems, yet we continue to send a growing number of prisoners, including many with serious mental disorders, to supermaximum security units. And we know that releasing prisoners from solitary confinement units straight into the community is likely to result in their failing to adjust and possibly committing violent crimes, yet we force a growing number of prisoners to "max out of the SHU" with little or no prerelease planning.

Why does our society continue to support the logic of law and order when it is so clearly designed to fail? Shifting momentarily to another area of public policy, Jonathan Kozol points out that our public schools are not failing, they are succeeding, but we have to realize that the job they are set up to do is not to provide all children with an access to education, but to track children, to train inner-city children to have low expectations, and to blame their own stupidity for their low station, while middle- and upper-class students are being prepared to succeed in college and beyond.

Similarly, the goals of the current imprisonment binge seem to have little to do with halting crime and "correcting" criminals. Quite the opposite! Prisons have become a very big business. And those who make huge profits from building and supplying correctional facilities, running private prisons, and investing in the prison industry grow richer when the prisons fail to correct or rehabilitate felons.

The entrenched interests that engineer prison expansion are certainly aware of the problems inherent in an increasingly brutal penal system. They know that denying mentally ill prisoners adequate psychiatric care and locking them in a SHU will make them more dangerous when they are released. Yet they keep on building new prisons and treating prisoners cruelly. Their intent is not difficult to fathom: They want to lock up even more people, for longer terms, which translates into more profits and power for them, even though they know that will not make our streets safer.

Of course, the public rarely thinks about such things. The silencing of all those who might move us to reconsider the trend toward harsher sentences has been so successful in recent years that any politician or judge who thinks about exposing the foolishness in current correctional policies has to worry about ruining her chances of ever winning another election.

But when we do give some thought to the contradictions, for instance the ones I have pointed out in regard to prisoners suffering from serious mental disorders, it is obvious that current correctional policies are designed to fail. Those who profit from that failure have the audacity to use the failures themselves—the growing rate of violence and mental breakdowns behind bars as well as the rising re-arrest rate among ex-prisoners—to rationalize our throwing even more money at the prisons!

## The Prison-Industrial Complex

The interlocking web of entrenched interests that profit from prison expansion constitute the Prison-Industrial Complex. To identify the key players, we merely need to ask who is happy when there are more prisons and more prisoners. There are at least seven obvious groups:

1. Politicians who use the rhetoric of law and order to gain votes, stay in office, and scare constituencies and fellow-politicians into supporting the kinds of laws they advocate; and the special interest groups that weave prison expansion into their agenda. The corporations that profit most from the expansion of our prison system are heavily represented among the large contributors to these politicians' campaign coffers.
2. The state and federal administrators and governmental agencies that control criminal justice and corrections and seek to expand their budgets as well as their influence. When there is violence in the prisons, and when ex-prisoners fail and have

to return to prison, their agencies and departments can justify requests for larger budgets.

3. Correctional employees. For example, the California Correctional Police Officers Association is one of the strongest unions and most important lobbies in California. Guards receive salaries in excess of $50,000 per year, and their union made the single largest contribution to the 1994 reelection campaign of law-and-order Governor Pete Wilson.
4. Private corporations and contractors who profit from the construction and operation of prisons, including the developers and contractors who build them and the suppliers who provide such things as food, uniforms, guns, and security equipment.
5. Private prison corporations who contract with states and counties to run correctional facilities for profit. For example, Corrections Corporation of America (CCA), a for-profit corporation that contracts with states to run correctional institutions, has ranked among the top five performing companies on the New York Stock Exchange for the past three years. The price of CCA stock climbed from $8 a share in 1992 to $30 in 1997. The value of all CCA shares grew from $50 million when the corporation went public in 1986 to over $3.5 billion in October 1997. And the corporation's revenue rose by 81 percent in 1995 alone. The more prisoners there are and the longer they stay, the greater the profits and the higher the stock. And of course, in order to enlarge their profits, these corporations reduce the level of security and mental health staffing and cut corners on drug rehabilitation, counseling, and literacy programs.
6. Private suppliers of prison health and mental health services. As in the case of managed care companies in the community, private suppliers have a financial incentive to provide fewer, more cost-effective services. If a prisoner is considered "bad"

and not "mad" and he is sent to a punitive lock-up unit, there is one less prisoner in need of psychiatric treatment.

7. For-profit companies that utilize prisoner labor. Many companies are figuring out that prisoners provide reliable labor at a very low wage. Prison rules prevent them from organizing and participating in collective bargaining, and the average pay to prisoners is 43 cents per hour. Prisoners are very willing to work, even for very low wages, because without the work they would be idle and broke.

While the imprisonment binge was expanding, various people and organizations figured out ways to wrangle profits and power out of the evolving phenomenon. The result is a Prison-Industrial Complex that feeds on its own failures to "correct" while growing and garnering immense profits at the expense of all other public services and priorities.

## The Economic Reality

There are many problems with the imprisonment binge, including the inhumanity in locking up and brutalizing so many people, the racism involved in confining a large segment of our young citizens of color, the unconstitutional and draconian measures that are necessary to carry out the plan, and the very dire consequences for people on the outside—the families and communities of prisoners as well as the rest of us.

Many people are so afraid of crime on the streets, so convinced of the need for revenge against criminals, and so inured to the prisoners' plight that they won't let logic and "humanistic" arguments deter their faith in the plan to lock 'em up and throw away the key. Perhaps, for them, it will be the economics of the situation that will eventually become compelling. While the crime rate is relatively flat, we continue to sink a growing proportion of scarce public funds into prisons at the expense of other important social programs such as schools and public health.

For example, California spent 3 percent of its state budget on prisons in 1980 and 18 percent on higher education. In 1994, the state spent 8 percent of its budget on prisons and 8 percent on higher education, and since 1994 spending on prisons has far exceeded spending on higher education. Nationwide spending on state prisons has risen faster than any other spending category in the last twenty years. In the same period, spending on elementary education, highways, welfare, and public health care have all diminished. The economic disaster does not end there. The U.S. Department of Justice admits that for every $100 million state legislatures spend on new prison construction, they are committing the taxpayers to spend $1.6 billion over the next three decades to operate the new facilities.

Obviously the logic of law and order is pure folly from an economic perspective. But if we are to transcend that "logic" and the accelerating imprisonment frenzy it rationalizes, we need an alternative plan.

## A Plan That Will Work

When it comes to criminal justice policy, we are at a fork in the road, and if we take the wrong path, it will be extremely difficult to turn back. If we continue to throw money at the prisons and send large sections of our low-income citizenry to be brutalized inside them, we are headed for social disaster. The people we consign to lives in prison will react to the denial of their humanity with outrage and resistance. There will be more rage, madness, and crime. Even harsher punishments will be devised. Each security innovation inside penal institutions will cost more, so a greater proportion of public moneys will have to be committed to imprisonment. The survivors of imprisonment will be less likely to succeed in their postrelease ventures and more will return to drugs and crime. The streets will be no safer, but the Prison-Industrial Complex will become such a powerful sector of our economy and our political landscape that it will defeat all opposition to its cynical plans.

As a result, there will be even fewer public resources for health care, education, child protective services, libraries, road maintenance, and so forth. As though envisioning just such a scenario, Andrew Young said on a visit to South Central Los Angeles following the disturbances that were set off by the acquittal of the officers who beat Rodney King: "You can't lock up enough men to have peace!"

---

Alternatively, if we refuse to carry out the logic of law and order to its tragic conclusion, we must take these steps to reverse the destructive imprisonment binge of recent years:

1. We have to break the silence about the horrors that occur in our prisons on a regular basis. We need to find out what is going on inside and go public with the bad news. We cannot permit the inhumanity and cruelty I have described in relation to mentally disordered felons to continue. The public must demand that the press be admitted to the prisons to interview prisoners and staff. Then the press and other media must be pressured to cover the story.

In addition, all branches of government need to launch investigations to determine why so many prisoners are suffering from serious mental disorders, why conditions in the jails and prisons are so harsh and inhumane, and what we can do to guarantee adequate mental health treatment. Citizens' review boards and adequately funded nonprofit prison legal aid and watchdog organizations need to be empowered to carry out concurrent investigations and make certain the government investigations are thorough and honest and result in significant reforms.

2. We have to assess the failures of our public mental health system outside prisons, and correct what ails that system while doing our best to keep individuals suffering from severe and persistent mental illnesses out of prison.

3. We have to change our attitudes about criminals—they are still human beings—and about the people we tend to criminalize, including the homeless, low-income people, immigrants, seriously mentally disordered individuals, and people of color. In terms of the criminalization of people with mental disorders, we need to reconsider the trend in the judicial system to give so little weight to the mental status of offenders in determining guilt and sentencing. I am not arguing they should all be exonerated, merely that consideration of their mental condition should lead to the diversion of a large proportion of defendants with histories of serious mental disorders into secure treatment programs.

4. We have to reform our prisons and change them into institutions that respect human life and the constitutional rights of all citizens. As I outline in Chapter Ten, the critical changes are reestablishment of meaningful education and rehabilitation programs, aggressive efforts to enrich the frequency and quality of visitation, an end to supermaximum security units and other forms of long-term lock-up and solitary confinement, and a concerted effort to maximize the fairness of disciplinary hearings and classification determinations. Of course, since mentally ill felons suffer an immense amount of pain and their disabilities worsen when they are left idle in overcrowded prisons and are sent to supermaximum security units, these reforms will greatly benefit mentally ill felons.

5. Since it is not possible to prevent entirely the incarceration of mentally ill felons, and since a certain number of prisoners will still be driven mad inside even if we correct the worst abuses in the prisons, we need to establish quality, comprehensive mental health treatment programs inside the prisons. I outline a plan to accomplish that in Chapter Ten.

6. We need to effect the changes in the criminal justice system I outline in Chapter Ten. High on the list of priorities is the diversion of people who have not committed serious or violent crimes, for instance those arrested for victimless drug-related crimes, to nonprison programs such as mandatory drug treatment in the community.

Also at the top of the list is the need to end racial disparity in sentencing and to reverse the pattern of longer and harsher sentences for people of color for almost every type of crime.

7. If there is to be substantial reform in our criminal justice system, we have to pay attention to the plight of those we have been ignoring. Instead of imprisoning people who live in poverty, we have to do all we can to end poverty, beginning with a serious attempt to reestablish the safety net we were strengthening during the "war on poverty" years.

As I mention in Chapter Ten, we can begin to attack social problems by attending to the problems of troubled youth. Researchers at Rand Corporation compared the costs and effectiveness of incarceration with the costs and benefits of early intervention programs for at-risk youth, and concluded that early intervention is more effective and less expensive than incarceration. We need to establish better educational and job-training programs in our inner cities. Why not invest more in young people on the front end—including counseling and community organizing projects to help them steer clear of drugs and gangs—in order to save a lot of money on incarceration at the back end?

Everyone I have spoken to who works with troubled youth—including ex-prisoners, who are impressively overrepresented among the ranks of counselors to troubled youth—reports that great gains are possible. Dedicated counselors in just about every low-income community in this country are trying to help young people understand that you can only eventually attain what you envision for yourself, so aim higher than death or prison.

Prison is an assault on the capacity to envision. Currently, all a prisoner sees in his future is steel bars, fights on the yard, and more secure and stark "holes." So why should he be motivated to go to classes or learn a trade? One African-American prisoner, who was repairing a rain-damaged wall when I interviewed him, said it succinctly: "A contractor ain't gonna hire a black ex-con with a drug record when there are so many white guys out there who are clean, looking for work in construction." So this man gives up the idea of ever bettering his situation. The worse the prison conditions, the less possibility there is for the prisoners to sustain a positive vision. Prisoners need to be helped to regain their reason to hope and their capacity to envision a productive future.

It is sheer folly to continue locking up a large number of people, brutalizing them, and throwing them into the same institutions as people who are suffering from serious mental disorders. Only by envisioning a society that solves its social problems as a whole, without "disappearing" a large number of its members and canceling their citizenship, can we proceed to enact a rational, cost-effective, and humane plan to run our prisons and to distribute mental health services to people who suffer from psychiatric disorders.

# Endnotes

## Preface

P. xv Deinstitutionalization: Lamb, R. H. "Improving Our Public Mental Health Systems." *Archives of General Psychiatry*, 1989, 4(6), 743–744; Bachrach, L. L. *An Overview of Deinstitutionalization*. New Directions for Mental Health Services. San Francisco: Jossey-Bass, 1993; Johnson, A. B. *Out of Bedlam: The Truth About Deinstitutionalization*. New York: Basic Books, 1991; and Shenson, D., Dubler, N., and Michaels, D. "Jails and Prisons: The New Asylums?" *American Journal of Public Health*, 1990, *80*(6), 655–656.

P. xix Willie's story: Corcoran, Kevin. "Sick Justice." *The Times* (Munster, Indiana), September 14, 1997.

P. xxi Prisons contain (statistics): U.S. Department of Justice, Bureau of Justice Statistics. "Sourcebook of Criminal Justice Statistics," online at http://www.albany.edu/sourcebook, 1996; Donziger, S. R. (ed.). *The Real War on Crime: The Report of the National Criminal Justice Commission*. New York: Harper Perennial, 1996.

P. xxii Rate of second arrests: Tonry, M. "President Clinton, Mandatory Minimums, and Disaffirmative Action." *Tikkun*, Nov./Dec., 1997.

P. xxv "Replacement effect": Hagan, J. "The Imprisoned Society: Time Turns a Classic on Its Head." *Sociological Forum*, 1995, *10*(3), 519–525.

P. xxvi Comparison of crime and imprisonment rates in the fifty states: Irwin, J., and Austin, J. *It's About Time: America's Imprisonment*

*Binge*. Belmont, California: Wadsworth, 1994; and Selke, W. L. *Prisons in Crisis*. Bloomington: Indiana University Press, 1993.

## Chapter One

P. 11 The prevalence of mental disorders: Steadman, H. J., Monahan, J., Harstone, E., et. al. "Mentally Disordered Offenders: A National Survey of Patients and Facilities." *Law and Human Behavior*, 1982, 6, 31–38; Smith, R. "How Many Mentally Abnormal Prisoners?" *British Medical Journal*, 1984, 288, 309–313; Norman & Cotton Associates, Young and Standard Consulting Corporation. *Current Description, Evaluation, and Recommendations for Treatment of Mentally Disordered Criminal Offenders*: Vol. 1, *Introduction and Prevalence (The Stirling Report)*. Sacramento: California Department of Corrections, Health Care Services, 1987; Teplin, L. A. "The Prevalence of Severe Mental Disorder Among Male Urban Jail Detainees: Comparison with the Epidemiologic Catchment Area Program." *American Journal of Public Health*, 1990, 80 (6), 663–669; Hodgins, S. "Assessing Mental Disorder in the Criminal Justice System: Feasibility Versus Clinical Accuracy." *International Journal of Law and Psychiatry*, 1995, 8(1), 15–28; Jemelka, R., Trupin, E., and Chiles, J. A. "The Mentally Ill in Prisons: A Review." *Hospital and Community Psychiatry*, 1989, 40(5), 481–491; Cote, G., and Hodgins, S. "Co-occurring Mental Disorders Among Criminal Offenders." *Bulletin American Academy of Psychiatry and Law*, 1990, 8(3), 271–281; Lamb, H. R., and Weinberger, L. E. "Persons with Severe Mental Illness in Jails and Prisons: A Review." *Psychiatric Services*, 1998, 49(4), 483–492.

P. 15 Breakdowns during incarceration: Toch, H. *Mosaic of Despair: Human Breakdowns in Prison*. Washington, D.C.: American Psychological Association, 1975, 1992; Cohen, S., and Taylor, L. *Psychological Survival: The Experience of Long-Term Imprisonment*. New York: Vintage, 1974.

P. 20 Aaron's story: "Inmate's Condition Deteriorates as Push for Appeal Drags On." *Houston Chronicle*, June 29, 1997.

P. 22 Women Prisoners (statistics): Bureau of Justice Statistics. *Women in Prison: Survey of State Prison Inmates*. Washington, D.C.: Bureau of Justice Statistics, 1991; E. Rosenblatt (ed.). *Criminal Injustice: Confronting the Prison Crisis*. Boston: South End Press, 1996, pp. 130–135.

P. 28 Testify: Kupers, T. Testimony in *Gates* v. *Deukmejian*, No. CIV. 2–87–1636–LKK. Reporter's Transcript of Proceedings, October 23, 1989, pp. 160–161.

P. 32 Goffman, E., *Asylums*. Garden City, N.Y.: Anchor Books, 1961; Scheff, T. *Being Mentally Ill: A Sociological Theory*. Chicago: Aldine, 1966.

## Chapter Two

P. 39 Early childhood trauma: Amaya-Jackson, L., and March, J. S. "Posttraumatic Stress Disorder in Children and Adolescents." *Child and Adolescent Psychiatric Clinics of North America*, Vol. 2: *Anxiety*, Philadelphia: Saunders, 1993, 639–654; Bell, C., and Jenkins, E. "Traumatic Stress and Children in Danger." *Journal of Health Care for the Poor and Underserved*, 1991, *2*, 175–185; Breslau, N., Davis, G. C., Andreski, P., and Peterson, E. "Traumatic Events and Posttraumatic Stress Disorder in an Urban Population of Young Adults." *Archives of General Psychiatry*, 1991, *48*, 216–222; Burton, D., Foy, D., Bwanausi, C., Johnson, J., and Moore, L. "The Relationship Between Traumatic Exposure, Family Dysfunction, and Post-traumatic Stress Symptoms in Male Juvenile Offenders." *Journal of Trauma Stress*, 1994, *7*, 83–93; Cooley-Quille, M., Turner, S., and Beidel, D. "Emotional Impact of Children's Exposure to Community Violence: A Preliminary Study." *Journal of the American Academy of Child and Adolescent Psychiatry*, 1995, *34*, 1362–1368; Garbarino, J., Kosteiny, K., and Dubrow, N. *No Place to Be a Child*. San Francisco: Jossey-Bass, 1991; Shakoor, and Debora, C. "Co-Victimization of African-American Children Who Witness Violence: Effects on Cognitive, Emotional and Behavioral Development." *Journal of the National Medical Association*, 1991, 83, 233–238.

P. 41 Massachusetts study: *Delinquent Youth and Family Violence: A Study of Abuse and Neglect in the Homes of Serious Juvenile Offenders*. Commonwealth of Massachusetts. Boston, Department of Youth Services, 1985.

P. 42 Link between trauma and criminal behavior: Collins, J., and Bailey, S. "Traumatic Stress Disorder and Violent Behavior." *Journal of Traumatic Stress*, 1990, *3*(2), 203–220; Steiner, H., Garcia, I. G., and Matthews, Z. "Posttraumatic Stress Disorder in Incarcerated Juvenile Delinquents." *Journal of the American Academy of Child and Adolescent Psychiatry*, 1997, *36*(3), 357–365; Kupers, T. A. "Trauma and Its Sequelae in Male Prisoners: Effects of Confinement, Overcrowding, and Diminished Services." *American Journal of Orthopsychiatry*, 1996, *66*(2), 189–196.

P. 47 Crowding: Calhoun, J. "Population Density and Social Pathology." *Science*, 1962, *206*, 139–148; D'Atri, D. "Psychophysiological Responses to Crowding." *Environment and Behavior*, 1975, *7*, 237–251; Ekland-Olson, S. "Crowding, Social Control, and Prison Violence: Evidence from the Post-Ruiz Years in Texas." *Law and Society Review*, 1986, 20, 289–421; Paulus, P. B., McCain, G., and Cox, V. C. "Death Rates, Psychiatric Commitments, Blood Pressure, and Perceived Crowding as a Function of Institutional Crowding." *Environmental Psychology and Nonverbal Behavior*, 1978, 3,107–117; Thornberry, T., and Call, J. "Constitutional Challenges to Prison Overcrowding: The Scientific Evidence of Harmful Effects." *Hastings Law Journal*, 1983, *35*, 313–353.

P. 57 The SHU Syndrome: Grassian, S. "Psychopathological Effects of Solitary Confinement." *American Journal of Psychiatry*, 1983, *140*(11), 1450–1454; Grassian, S., and Friedman, N. "Effects of Sensory Deprivation in Psychiatric Seclusion and Solitary Confinement." *International Journal of Law and Psychiatry*, 1986, 8, 49–65; Hodgins, S., and Cote, G. "The Mental Health of Penitentiary Inmates in Isolation." *Canadian Journal of Criminology*, 1991, 175–182.

P. 57 Women housed in supermaximum control units: Korn, R. Excerpts from a report on the effects of confinement in the Lexington High

Security Unit. In Churchill, W., and Vander Wall, J. J. (eds.). *Cages of Steel: The Politics of Imprisonment in the United States*. Washington, D.C.: Maisonneuve Press, 1992, pp. 123–127.

P. 58 40 percent are functionally illiterate: The Center on Crime, Communities, and Culture. "Education as Crime Prevention." *Research Brief, Occasional Paper Series*, September 1997, Vol. 2. New York: Center on Crime, Communities, and Culture (888 Seventh Ave., NY, NY 10106).

## Chapter Three

P. 65 Declaration: Kupers, T. *Coleman* v. *Wilson*, No. CIV S 90–0520 LKK-JFM, February 16, 1993. U.S. District Court, Eastern District of California, Ninth Circuit.

P. 68 Standards: National Commission on Correctional Health Care. *Standards for Health Services in Prisons*. Chicago: National Commission on Correctional Health Care, 1997; American Psychiatric Association, *Psychiatric Services in Jails and Prisons*. APA Task Force Report. Washington, D.C.: American Psychiatric Association, 1989; American Public Health Association, *Standards for Health Services in Prisons*. Washington, D.C.: USPHA, 1986.

P. 79 Suicide: Smialek, J., and Spitz, W. "Death Behind Bars." *Journal of the American Medical Association*, 1978, *240*, 256370–256371.

P. 85 Burnout: Maslach, C., and Leiter, M. P. *The Truth About Burnout: How Organizations Cause Personal Stress and What to Do About It*. San Francisco: Jossey-Bass, 1997.

## Chapter Four

P. 94 Racial disparity in sentencing: Petersilia, J. "Racial Disparities in the Criminal Justice System." Prepared for the National Institute of Corrections, U.S. Department of Justice (R–2947–NIC), by the Rand Corporation, 1983; Mauer, M. "Young Black Americans and the Criminal Justice System: Five Years Later." Washington, D.C.: The Sentencing Project, 1995; Donziger, S. (Ed). *The Real War on Crime: The Report of the National Criminal Justice Commission*. New

York: Harper/Collins, 1996; Miller, J. G. *Search and Destroy: African-American Males in the Criminal Justice System*. New York: Cambridge University Press, 1996; Davidson, J. "Caged Cargo: African-Americans Are Grist for the Fast-Growing Prison Industry's Money Mill." *Emerge*, October, 1997, 36–46.

P. 98 Human Rights Watch team: Human Rights Watch. *Cold Storage: Super-Maximum Security Confinement in Indiana*. New York: Human Rights Watch, 1997.

P. 99 Prison gang-containment policies: Kassel, P. The Gang Crackdown in Massachusetts' Prisons: Arbitrary and Harsh Treatment Can Only Make Matters Worse." *New England Journal on Criminal and Civil Confinement*, 1998, *24*, 1, 37–63.

P. 101 One inmate gladiator: Weinstein, C. "Brutality at Corcoran." *Prison Focus*, 1997, *1*(1), 4–5.

P. 104 Lease black convicts: Oshinsky, D. M. *Worse Than Slavery: Parchman Farm and the Ordeal of Jim Crow Justice*. New York: The Free Press, 1996.

P. 107 O'Neil Stough. Personal communication, 1997.

P. 111 California study: cited in Donziger (1996), p. 120.

### Chapter Five

P. 113 Reasons they are incarcerated (statistics): Bureau of Justice Statistics. *Women in Prison: Survey of State Prison Inmates*. Washington, D.C.: Bureau of Justice Statistics, 1991; E. Rosenblatt (ed.). *Criminal Injustice: Confronting the Prison Crisis*. Boston: South End Press, 1996, pp. 130–135; Bloom, B. "Tracking the Population Explosion." *The Women's Review of Books*, 1997, *14*(10–11), 7.

P. 114 Depression in women prisoners: Velimesis, M. L. "Sex Roles and Mental Health of Women in Prison." *Professional Psychology*, 1981, *12*(1), 128–135; Policy Research Associates. "The Mental Health Services Needs of Women in the Criminal Justice System." Report to the National Institute of Justice, Washington, D.C., October, 1994.

P. 117 Geraldine: "Breaking the Cycle: Two Ex-Convicts Talk about Life In and Out of Prison." *The Women's Review of Books*, 1997, 14(10–11), 12–13.

P. 126 Bentham's "Panopticon": Foucault, M. *Discipline and Punish: The Birth of the Prison*. New York: Pantheon, 1977.

P. 131 Complex PTSD: Herman, J. *Trauma and Recovery: The Aftermath of Violence—from Domestic Abuse to Political Terror*. New York: Basic Books, 1992.

## Chapter Six

P. 137 The incidence of rape among men: Lockwood, D. *Prison Sexual Violence*. New York: Elsevier North Holland, Inc., 1980; Stuckman-Johnson, S., et. al. (1996). "Sexual Coercion Reported by Men and Women in Prison." *The Journal of Sex Research*, 33(1),67–76.

P. 137 The incidence of rape of women prisoners: Human Rights Watch. "Sexual Abuse of Women Prisoners in the U.S." In *The Human Rights Watch Global Report on Women's Human Rights*. New York: Human Rights Watch, 1995, pp. 156–182; Human Rights Watch. *All Too Familiar: Sexual Abuse of Women in U.S. State Prisons*. New York: Human Rights Watch, 1996.

P. 140 Suffolk County incident: Hodges, M. "Prison Rape." *Out*, March, 1998.

P. 142 James Dunn story: Rideau, W. "The Sexual Jungle." In W. Rideau and R. Wikberg (eds.), *Life Sentences: Rage and Survival Behind Bars*. New York: Times Books, 1992, pp. 73–107.

P. 143 Stop Prisoner Rape: Donaldson, D. Op-Ed: "The Rape Crisis Behind Bars." *New York Times*, December 1993. Or contact Stop Prisoner Rape, P.O. Box 286, Village Station, New York, NY 10014.

P. 144 Zelda's story: Human Rights Watch. "Sexual Abuse of Women Prisoners in the U.S. in *The Human Rights Watch Global Report on Women's Human Rights*. New York: Human Rights Watch, 1995, p. 165.

P. 147 Dublin, California incident: *San Francisco Examiner*, September 29, 1996.

P. 152 HIV and AIDS: Braithwaite, R. L., Hammett, T. M., and Mayberry, R. M. *Prisons and AIDS: A Public Health Challenge*. San Francisco: Jossey-Bass, 1996; Polych, C. "Punishment within Punishment: The AIDS Epidemic in North American Prisons." *Men's Studies Review*, 1992, 9, 13–17.

## Chapter Seven

P. 157 Research shows that continuous contact: Holt, N., and Miller, D. *Explorations in Inmate-Family Relationships*. Sacramento: California Department of Corrections, Research Report No. 46; 1972; Jorgensen, J. D., Hernandez, S. H., and Warren, R. C. "Addressing the Social Needs of Families of Prisoners: A Tool for Inmate Rehabilitation." *Federal Probation*, 1986, 38, 47–52.

P. 158 Research involving visitation and recidivism: Holt, N., and Miller, D. *Explorations in Inmate-Family Relationships*. Sacramento: California Department of Corrections, Research Report No. 46; 1972; Kupers, T. "Contact Between the Bars: A Rationale for Consultation in Prisons." *Urban Health*, 1976, 5, 38–39.

P. 159 California's Family Visiting Program: Glaser, D. *Preparing Convicts for Law-Abiding Lives: The Pioneering Penology of Richard A. McGee*. Albany, New York: State University of New York Press, 1995, pp. 71–74.

P. 164 Bus therapy: Martin, D. M. and Sussman, P. Y. *Committing Journalism: The Prison Writings of Red Hog*. New York: Norton, 1993.

P. 167 A prisoner and his mother: Transcript of trial (November 10, 1983, pp. 435–548), *Toussaint* v. *McCarthy*, 597 F. Supp. 1388, 1393, Ninth Circuit, 1984.

## Chapter Eight

P. 176 Suicide in jails: Smialek, J., and Spitz, W. "Death Behind Bars." *Journal of the American Medical Association*, 1978, 240, 256370–256371; Hayes, L., and Kajdan, B. *Final Report to the*

*National Institute of Corrections on the National Study of Jail Suicides*. Washington, D.C.: The National Center on Institutions and Alternatives, 1981; Hayes, L. "National Study of Jail Suicides: Seven Years Later." *Psychiatric Quarterly*, 1989, 60(1), Spring; Hayes, L. *Prison Suicide: An Overview and Guide to Prevention*. Washington, D.C.: National Institute of Corrections, U.S. Department of Justice, June, 1995; B. Danto (ed.). *Jail House Blues*. Orchard Lake, Michigan: Epic Publications, 1973.

P. 177 Suicide in prisons: Hayes, L. *Prison Suicide: An Overview and Guide to Prevention*. Washington, D.C.: National Institute of Corrections, U.S. Department of Justice, grant No. 93P01GHU1, June, 1995; Liebling, A. *Suicides in Prison*. London: Routledge, 1992.

## Chapter Nine

P. 197 Frank "Big Black" Smith's case: *Prison Legal News*, November, 1997.

P. 205 Research on institutional dynamics: Haney, C., Banks, C., and Zimbardo, P. G. "Interpersonal Dynamics in a Simulated Prison." *International Journal of Criminology and Penology*, 1973, *1*, 69–97.

P. 207 Indiana's Maximum Control Facility: Human Rights Watch, *Cold Storage: Super-Maximum Security Confinement in Indiana*. New York: Human Rights Watch, 1997.

## Chapter Ten

P. 220 Minimum standards for correctional health care: National Commission on Correctional Health Care. *Standards for Health Services in Prisons*. Chicago: National Commission on Correctional Health Care, 1997; American Psychiatric Association, *Psychiatric Services in Jails and Prisons*. APA Task Force Report. Washington, D.C.: American Psychiatric Association, 1989; American Public Health Association. *Standards for Health Services in Prisons*. Washington, D.C.: USPHA, 1986.

P. 220 "Written policy and defined procedures. . . .": National Commission on Correctional Health Care. *Standards for Health Services in*

*Prisons*. Chicago: National Commission on Correctional Health Care, 1997, p. 38.

P. 222 We know how to prevent suicides: Hayes, L. *Prison Suicide: An Overview and Guide to Prevention*. Washington, D.C.: National Institute of Corrections, U.S. Department of Justice, grant No. 93P01GHU1, June, 1995.

P. 226 Psychiatric Rehabilitation Programs: Anthony, W. A., and Liberman, R. P. "The Practice of Psychiatric Rehabilitation: Historical, Conceptual, and Research Base." *Schizophrenia Bulletin*, 1986, *12*(4), 542–559.

P. 227 Hans Toch's term for these felons: "Disturbed, Disruptive": Toch, H. *Corrections: A Humanistic Approach*. Guilderland, New York: Harrow and Heston, 1997.

P. 237 The presence of serious education programs in prison: The Center on Crime, Communities and Culture. *Education as Crime Prevention*. Research Brief, Occasional Paper Series, Vol. 2, 888 Seventh Ave., New York, New York 10106, September, 1997; Siegel, G. R. "A Research Study to Determine the Effect of Literacy and General Educational Development Programs on Adult Offenders on Probation." Tucson, Arizona: Adult Probation Department for the Superior Court in Pima County, 1997; Molitor, G. T. "Should Prison Inmates Receive Education Benefits?" *On the Horizon*, 1994, *2*(3), 9–10.

P. 237 The efficacy of general prison rehabilitation programs: Martinson, R. "What Works? Questions and Answers About Prison Reform." *Public Interest*, 1974, *3*(5), 22–54; Martinson, R. "New Findings, New Views: A Note of Caution Regarding Sentencing Reform." *Hofstra Law Review*, 1979, *7*(2), 243–258; Gendreau, P., and Ross, R. "Effective Correctional Treatment: Bibliotherapy for Cynics." *Crime and Delinquency*, 1979, *25*, 463–489, 1979; Palmer, T. "The Effectiveness of Intervention: Recent Trends and Current Issues." *Crime and Delinquency*, 1991, *37*(3), 330–346.

P. 241 Dr. Lige Dailey: Dailey, L. "Re-entry: Prospects for Postrelease Success." In D. Sabo, T. Kupers, and W. London (eds.), *Confronting*

*Prison Masculinities: The Gendered Politics of Punishment*. Philadelphia: Temple University Press, 1999, forthcoming.

P. 243 Create smaller facilities: Many people have suggested this concept, but Steve Martin was the first to explain to me its benefits (Personal communication).

P. 244 The National Criminal Justice Commission: see Donziger (1996); Irwin and Austin (1994); Jerome Miller (1996).

P. 245 Create alternatives for offenders: National Coalition for Mental and Substance Abuse Health Care in the Justice System. *Community Corrections in America: New Directions and Sounder Investments for Persons with Mental Illness and Codisorders*. Seattle, Washington: The National Coalition for Mental and Substance Abuse Health Care in the Justice System, 1905 Seventh Ave. West, March, 1996.

P. 252 Kathy Boudin. "Lessons from a Mother's Program in Prison: A Psychosocial Approach Supports Women and Their Children." *Women and Therapy*, 1998, *21*(1), 103–126.

P. 252 Santa Cruz Women's Project: Karlene Faith. "The Politics of Confinement and Resistance." In Rosenblatt, E. (ed.). *Criminal Injustice: Confronting the Prison Crisis*. Boston: South End Press, pp. 165–183.

P. 253Washington State Department of Corrections: Lovell, D., Rhodes, L., Dunnington, D., and Wilson, T. "Mobile Consultation: Sowing New Seeds in the Prison Culture." In Allen, D., (ed.). *Correctional Mental Health Collaboration*. Seattle, Washington: University of Washington Correctional Mental Health Collaboration, 1995.

P. 254 Worldwide Models: reviewed in Selke, W. I. *Prisons in Crisis*. Bloomington and Indianapolis: Indiana University Press, 1993.

## Chapter Eleven

P. 261 "The great secret. . . .": Menninger, K. *The Crime of Punishment*. New York: Viking, 1966, p. 190.

P. 266 Prison-Industrial Complex: Donziger, S. (ed.). *The Real War on Crime: The Report of the National Criminal Justice Commission*. New

York: Harper/Collins, 1996; Miller, J. G. *Search and Destroy: African-American Males in the Criminal Justice System*. New York: Cambridge University Press, 1996; Davis, Angela Y. "Race, Gender, and Prison History: From the Convict Lease System to the Supermax Prison." In D. Sabo, T. Kupers, and W. London (eds.), *Confronting Prison Masculinities: The Gendered Politics of Punishment*. Philadelphia: Temple University Press, 1999, forthcoming.

P. 267 Private prison corporations: Silverstein, K. "America's Private Gulag." *Prison Legal News*, 1997, 8(6),1–4; and Bates, E. "Private Prisons." *The Nation*, January 5, 1998, 11–18.

P. 268 For-profit companies that utilize prisoner labor: Parenti, C. "Making Prisons Pay." *The Nation*, January 29, 1996, 11–14.

P. 269 The economic disaster does not end there: See Donziger (1996).

P. 270 Young, A. In *The Fire This Time*. A film by Randy Holland. Los Angeles: Blacktop Films, 1994.

P. 272 Researchers at Rand Corporation: Greenwood, P. W. *Diverting Children from a Life of Crime: Measuring Costs and Benefits*. Santa Monica, California: Rand Corporation, 1996.

# For Further Reading


Abbott, J. H. *In the Belly of the Beast: Letters from Prison*. New York: Vintage, 1982.

Abu-Jamal, M. *Live from Death Row*. New York: Addison-Wesley, 1995.

Braithwaite, R. L., Hammett, T. M., and Mayberry, R. M. *Prisons and AIDS: A Public Health Challenge*. San Francisco: Jossey-Bass, 1996.

Churchill, W., and Vander Wall, J. J. (eds.). *Cages of Steel: The Politics of Imprisonment in the United States*. Washington, D. C.: Maisonneuve Press, 1992.

Cohen, S., and Taylor, L. *Psychological Survival: The Experience of Long-Term Imprisonment*. New York: Vintage, 1972.

Currie, E. *Confronting Crime: An American Challenge*. New York: Pantheon, 1985.

Currie, E. *Reckoning: Drugs, the Cities and the American Future*. New York: Hill and Wang, 1994.

Daly, K. *Gender, Crime and Punishment*. New Haven, Connecticut: Yale University Press, 1994.

Denborough, D. (ed.). *Beyond the Prison: Gathering Dreams of Freedom*. Adelaide, South Australia: Dulwich Centre Publications, 1996.

Donziger, S. (ed.). *The Real War on Crime: The Report of the National Criminal Justice Commission*. New York: Harper/Collins, 1996.

Faith, K. *Unruly Women: The Politics of Confinement and Resistance*. Vancouver, B.C.: Press Gang, 1993.

Feinman, C. *Women in the Criminal Justice System*. Westport, Connecticut: Praeger, 1994.

Foucault, M. *Discipline and Punish: The Birth of the Prison*. New York: Pantheon, 1977.

Gilligan, J. *Violence: Our Deadly Epidemic and Its Causes*. New York: Grosset/Putnam, 1996.

Glaser, D. *Preparing Convicts for Law-abiding Lives: The Pioneering Penology of Richard A. McGee*. Albany, New York: State University of New York Press, 1995.

Goffman, E. *Asylums: Essays on the Social Situation of Mental Patients and Other Inmates*. New York: Doubleday, Anchor, 1961.

Halleck, S. L. *Psychiatry and the Dilemmas of Crime: A Study of Causes, Punishment, and Treatment*. New York: Harper and Row, 1967.

Herman, J. *Trauma and Recovery: The Aftermath of Violence—From Domestic Abuse to Political Terror*. New York: Basic Books, 1992.

Human Rights Watch. "Sexual Abuse of Women Prisoners in the U.S." In *The Human Rights Watch Global Report on Women's Human Rights*. New York: Human Rights Watch, 1995.

Human Rights Watch. *All Too Familiar: Sexual Abuse of Women in U.S. State Prisons*. New York: Human Rights Watch, 1996.

Human Rights Watch. *Cold Storage: Super-Maximum Security Confinement in Indiana*. New York: Human Rights Watch, 1997.

Irwin, J. *The Felon*. Englewood Cliffs, New Jersey: Prentice-Hall, 1970.

Irwin, J., and Austin, J. *It's About Time: America's Imprisonment Binge*. Belmont, California: Wadsworth, 1994.

Jacobs, J. *Stateville*. Chicago: University of Chicago Press, 1977.

Johnson, A. B. *Out of Bedlam: The Truth About Deinstitutionalization*. New York: Basic Books, 1990.

Martin, D. M., and Sussman, P. Y. *Committing Journalism: The Prison Writings of Red Hog*. New York: Norton, 1993.

Mauer, M., and Huling, T. *Young Black Americans and the Criminal Justice System: Five Years Later*. Washington, D.C.: The Sentencing Project, 1995.

Mauer, M., and Young, M. C. *Truths, Half-Truths, and Lies: Myths and Realities About Crime and Punishment*. Washington, D.C.: The Sentencing Project, 1996.

Menninger, K. *The Crime of Punishment*. New York: Vintage, 1969.

Miller, J. G. *Search and Destroy: African-American Males in the Criminal Justice System*. New York: Cambridge University Press, 1996.

Pollock-Byrne, J. *Women, Prison and Crime*. Pacific Grove, California: Brooks/Cole, 1990.

Prejean, H. *Dead Man Walking*. New York: Vintage, 1993.

*Prison Focus*. Quarterly publication of California Prison Focus, 2489 Mission Street, Suite 28, San Francisco, CA 94110.

*Prison Legal News*. Monthly publication, 2400 N.W. 80th Street, Suite 148, Seattle, WA 98117.

Rideau, W., and Wikberg, R. *Life Sentences: Rage and Survival Behind Bars*. New York: Times Books, 1992.

Rierden, A. *The Farm: Life Inside a Women's Prison*. Amherst: University of Massachusetts Press, 1997.

Rosenblatt, E. (ed.). *Criminal Injustice: Confronting the Prison Crisis*. Boston: South End Press, 1996.

Rothman, D. *The Discovery of the Asylum*. Boston: Little, Brown, 1971.

Rothman, D. *Conscience and Convenience: The Asylum and Its Alternatives in Progressive America*. Boston: Little, Brown, 1980.

Sabo, D., Kupers, T., and London, W. *Confronting Prison Masculinities: The Gendered Politics of Punishment*. Philadelphia: Temple University Press, 1999, forthcoming.

Scacco, A. *Rape in Prison*. Springfield: Thomas, 1975.

Selke, W. I. *Prisons in Crisis*. Bloomington and Indianapolis: Indiana University Press, 1993.

Shapiro-Bertolini, E. *Through the Walls: Prison Correspondence*. Culver City, California: Peace Press, 1976.

Toch, H. *Mosaic of Despair: Human Breakdowns in Prison*. Washington, D.C.: American Psychological Association, 1975, 1992.

Toch, H. *Corrections: A Humanistic Approach*. Guilderland, New York: Harrow and Heston, 1997.

Tonry, M. *Malign Neglect: Race, Crime and Punishment in America*. New York: Oxford University Press, 1995.

# About the Author

Terry A. Kupers practices psychiatry in Oakland, California and teaches in the Graduate School of Psychology of the Wright Institute in Berkeley. He is a fellow of the American Psychiatric Association, president of the East Bay Psychiatric Association, and a member of California Psychiatric Association's Task Force on Corrections. He is co-chair of the Committee on the Mentally Ill Behind Bars of the American Association of Community Psychiatrists. He has served as a psychiatric expert in more than a dozen class action lawsuits concerning the conditions of confinement and the adequacy of mental health services in jails and prisons, and as consultant to the Civil Rights Division of the U.S. Department of Justice and to Human Rights Watch.

He is the author of *Public Therapy: The Practice of Psychotherapy in the Public Mental Health Clinic* (Free Press, 1981), *Ending Therapy: The Meaning of Termination* (New York University Press, 1988), and *Revisioning Men's Lives: Gender, Intimacy, and Power* (Guilford, 1993). He is a co-editor with Don Sabo and Willie London of *Confronting Prison Masculinities: The Gendered Politics of Punishment* (Temple University Press, 1999, forthcoming). He has written many professional articles and book chapters on a variety of topics.

Terry Kupers has worked and taught in several public mental health agencies and universities. He is married and has three sons.

# About the Author